# 2 Week WEIGHT LOSS Program

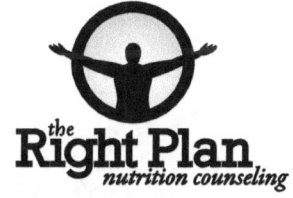

the
Right Plan
nutrition counseling

Name: Kellie Hill, NTP
ISBN-1500746401
ISBN-9781500746407

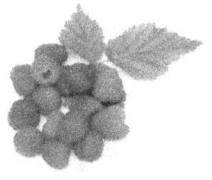

## DEDICATION

*To my loving husband for supporting my dreams and goals.*

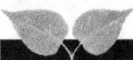

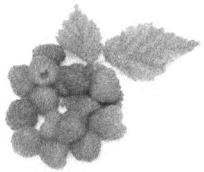

## ACKNOWLEDGEMENT

So many people have helped in this project that it would be another whole book for the full list. I might not remember everyone and I'm sorry if I forgot to mention you. Nothing is ever accomplished in a vacuum and those that have been my support system are many. Thanks to Doug Hill, Paradux Media Group, and my clients for inspiration.

**ALSO BY KELLIE HILL**
*Cleanse and Detoxify Your Body:*
*28 days to better health using nutrient dense whole foods*
http://www.amazon.com/dp/B00EKTP5AC

# TABLE OF CONTENTS

Meal Plans ................................................................. 23

Recipes: Dressings ...................................................... 39

Recipes: Breakfasts ..................................................... 45

Recipes: Snacks .......................................................... 55

Recipes: Lunches ........................................................ 65

Recipes: Dinners ......................................................... 75

Recipes: Side Dishes .................................................... 93

Recipes: Desserts ........................................................ 115

Recipe Index .............................................................. 123

About The Author ........................................................ 125

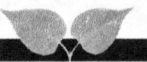

# WHY A WEIGHT LOSS PROGRAM?

As any of my clients can attest, I don't focus on strictly weight loss. My area of expertise is whole foods nutrition. A by-product of getting healthy frequently is losing weight. But, weight can be lost in an unhealthy manner compromising health. So, I originally chose not to focus on weight loss.

Then a few years ago one of my clients seemed to be doing everything right but her weight was stagnant above an ideal amount. We needed to "jump start" her metabolism in a healthy way. I created the original 2 Week Weight Loss Program. It wasn't meant to be a permanent diet but to get her over a hurdle and back on the right path. It worked brilliantly. She lost 10 pounds and had more energy. I don't recommend that fast of weight loss for anyone, but it showed her metabolism had become sluggish.

Soon I was frequently providing this plan to women and men interested in losing weight and having unlimited energy. Any time someone wanted to lose weight quickly, safely, and in a healthy fashion, I handed them a version of the 2 Week Weight Loss Program. And, many have come back to the program whenever they have important events, want to drop a few pounds, or just rev up their metabolism.

Over the years I have refined and changed the program for various clients with 100% success. It's a clear plan to help any one kick-start their personal plan or be ready for a big event.

Want extra motivation during these two weeks? No problem; I'm here to help. Subscribe at www.2WeekWeightLossProgram.com/Inspire and each day I'll send you a positive affirmation to keep you inspired and help you reach your goals.

## SUSAN'S STORY – I Lost 17 lbs. Without Trying

*Susan began nutritional therapy because she wanted to feel better. She wasn't sure the foods she was eating were helping her. Using the 2 Week Weight Loss Program we revved up her metabolism and eliminated foods that were decreasing her energy level. "I truly feel better eating foods wisely. It has been a wonderful learning experience. The bonus – I have lost 17 pounds without trying." Susan has continued to lose weight by adhering to the basic principles in the 2 Week Weight Loss Program. And she feels like she hasn't missed out on any life moments because of food. Her energy levels are consistent throughout the day allowing her to work all day and now, with this additional energy, she has begun a workout program as well; something she never could have done before.*

## WEIGHT LOSS WITH WHOLE FOODS VS. SUPPLEMENTS

The program is best completed as a whole foods diet. Everything in the meal plan can be purchased from traditional grocery stores, health food stores, or online. It includes three meals a day, two snacks a day, and a dessert. You will never feel hungry because you will eat as much as you desire of some of the foods.

For some people, making this many meals and snacks is overwhelming, even for only two weeks. In this case the two snacks a day can be replaced by a protein shake. This is a more convenient alternative for some. Two products I recommend are HealthForce Warrior Food or Garden of Life Raw Meal.

Either way, the 2 Week Weight Loss Program continues to have proven success.

### KIRSTEN'S STORY — I'm Below 20% Body Fat

*Kirsten had been a client for over a year when she wanted to fit into a particular pair of pants for her birthday celebration. The 2 Week Weight Loss Program was the answer. She tried it for the first week, losing 5 pounds. But, as a busy self-employed mother, wife, and community volunteer, she was finding it difficult to prepare all the snacks. "The food was tasty but I just didn't want to take the time to make the snacks. I began to feel time stress even though I was seeing results." Kirsten continued the program but substituted a protein shake in place of the whole food snacks. She lost another 4 pounds the second week. "The shake made the program a lot easier for me. The results were fantastic and continue to be." She has maintained below 20% body fat.*

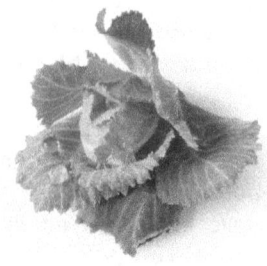

# IS THIS 2 WEEKS RIGHT FOR YOU?

There are a large variety of diet plans on the market, and almost all of them work for somebody. In fact you probably know someone who was successful on a particular diet plan; and you probably know someone who failed on the exact same diet plan. Many of these programs are very convenient with prepackaged meals ready to go. But, most are expensive and aren't focused on creating and maintaining overall health. The end result is just the number on the scale.

The 2 Week Weight Loss Program is designed to keep you healthy while you lose weight. No muscle will be cannibalized in order to lose weight. You won't feel hungry or deprived. You will have more energy, think clearer, feel better, and lose weight. These two weeks are designed to increase your metabolism so you'll look AND feel great.

This program is not for you if you aren't willing to cook. This is a whole foods diet plan, which means there aren't any boxes and few cans or jars to purchase. You will be spending time in your kitchen making your meals and snacks. Most of the meals and snacks are easy to prepare and leftovers are used to help save time.  If you don't have time to make all the foods, consider purchasing a protein shake to use in place of snacks.

For best results, start the 2 Week Weight Loss Program when you don't have multiple lunch or dinner meetings, plans for nights out at restaurants, etc. For two weeks you will need to focus on your food choices. In the overall years of life, fourteen days is nothing. But, if you can't commit to fourteen days for yourself, realize your results will vary from the normal weight loss.

The 2 Week Weight Loss Program is gluten free, low sugar, and mostly dairy free. The few recipes that include cheese can easily be made without cheese to accommodate lactose intolerance. Most importantly the two weeks includes few starchy carbohydrates and many high fiber foods along with high quality meats and good quality fats.

This program doesn't include an entire cookbook of recipes, just the two weeks. You also won't find different recipes for all 84 eating occasions. Although you will be preparing foods, I've tried to use your time efficiently by making multiple servings when possible and repeating the easiest snacks and desserts.

# WHEN AND HOW YOU EAT

For optimal results, your diet is more than just what you eat. Definitely what you put into your body is the most significant factor to your success, but it's not the only factor.

When you eat is important for speedy weight loss. Your metabolism needs to stay revved throughout the day to burn the most calories. In the 2 Week Weight Loss Program you will accomplish this by eating smaller meals more frequently. Even if you're not hungry, eat a few bites. This will keep your digestive system busy, your metabolism burning, and keep you from getting overly hungry later in the day. Space your meals and snacks for every few hours depending on the number of hours you will be awake.

For example, eat breakfast within 30 minutes of waking, let's say 6:30 a.m. First snack will be around 8:30 or 9 a.m. Lunch at 11:30 or noon. Second snack around 3 p.m. Dinner and dessert at 6 p.m. Bed at 10 p.m. This is just a rough idea. Don't go longer than 3 hours between eating in order to keep your metabolism burning and ensure weight loss. Don't eat later than two hours prior to bed so your food will be mostly digested before sleeping (when digestion and metabolism slow down).

How you eat is also important for speedy weight loss. The body needs to be in a parasympathetic state in order to properly digest food. You really can easily make this happen. Sit down to eat. Take a few deep breaths to unwind. Study the food you are about to eat – the look and the smell. Focus on eating, even if it's only a ten minute break. Study the taste and the texture. Don't watch television, work on the computer, read a book, etc. Focus! Remember, you have goals you want to attain. Plus you will be modeling amazingly healthy techniques for your children. Eat slowly and chew every bite as long as you can. There's a saying that for the best digestion we should drink our foods and chew our liquids – see if you can make that happen. If you need help slowing down, try eating with your non-dominate hand or putting your fork down between bites.

# UNDERSTANDING CARBOHYDRATES

I don't know if it's fair to state there are good and bad carbohydrates, but it's true there are better and worse ones when it comes to weight loss. In the 2 Week Weight Loss Program you will eliminate most of the less healthy carbohydrates that have a tendency to "plump" people up rather than slim them down. Yes, this means no bread, no alcohol, no pasta, and almost no sugar. It really isn't as bad as it sounds though, I promise.

All carbohydrates break down to sugar in our bodies, which is one of the primary fuels for energy. This is the reason why no-carb diets frequently fail because our body needs the fuel of carbohydrates, but it needs fuel that is long burning. The faster carbohydrates are processed and absorbed, generally speaking, the less healthy they are and the more likely they will be stored as fat on the body.

In the 2 Week Weight Loss Program I've chosen healthier carbohydrates that include fiber to slow digestion and clean the digestive tract. To that I've added good quality fats to continue slowing sugar absorption while keeping the gall bladder active.

## KERRI'S STORY — Healthy Choices A Natural Now

*"While there is no shortage of information regarding weight loss and nutrition out there, it can be overwhelming sorting through it all. Since becoming a client at The Right Plan I have been able to conquer the confusion and make healthy choices a natural part of my day. Kellie has shown me nutritious foods that I never, ever, imagined I would eat that have become a regular staple in our house. I actually love to grocery shop now and I am proud to say there is virtually no processed food in my house. I lost weight and kept it off during a very stressful time in my life." Kerri*

# NOT ALL FATS ARE CREATED EQUAL

Fat has been demonized. But some fats have a necessary place in all diets, including for weight loss. Fat provides most of the energy needed to perform much of the body's work, especially muscular work. Padding fats protect the internal organs from shock. Insulation fats protect against temperature extremes. In foods, nutrient fats provide essential fatty acids and transport fats carry fat-soluble vitamins (vitamins A, E, D, & K are not absorbed without fat). Fat contributes to feelings of fullness, aids in the absorption of some phytochemicals, and helps make foods tender. The key is to find the balance between what fat the body needs and what fat will harm the body.

A quick primer regarding fats: Saturated fats are highly stable so they are less likely to go rancid when heated during cooking. They are good for high heat cooking, such as roasting. Monounsaturated fats are relatively stable so they can be used in cooking at lower temperatures such as a quick sauté. Polyunsaturated fats are highly reactive when exposed to heat or oxygen and should never be heated. Additionally, the high heats and oxidation required to extract and process these oils can make them dangerous in the body. It is best to avoid highly industrially processed polyunsaturated oils such as corn, canola, cottonseed, and soy. Trans fats are a type of fat molecule produced by a process called "partial hydrogenation" which rearranges the hydrogen atoms in liquid unsaturated fatty acids to produce an unnatural fat which is solid at room temperature. Due to the chaos caused in our body by the unnatural trans fats they are highly dangerous and should be avoided completely.

In the 2 Week Weight Loss Program, I primarily use the saturated fat coconut oil and the monounsaturated fat extra virgin olive oil.

I know some people are afraid of the words "saturated fat" since it has become synonymous with "heart disease". But, there is a difference between the medium chain saturated fatty acids in coconut oil and the long chain fatty acids in other saturated fats. Coconut oil, because it is primarily made of medium and short-chain fatty acids, is broken down and used for energy production and seldom ends up as body fat or deposits in the arteries. It produces energy, not fat. It also has a negative effect on blood cholesterol and helps protect against heart disease.

# WHAT, HOW MUCH, & WHEN TO DRINK

What you drink is very important because it requires very little digestion and goes directly into your blood stream. If it's a sugary beverage it will cause an insulin surge. Most likely these calories will be stored as excess weight (unless you're in the middle of running a marathon) and you will be craving more sugar later. This includes sodas, energy drinks, fruit juices, alcohol, milk, etc.

Many busy people are not willing to give up caffeine, and I understand because I have my moments too. If you have the wherewithal, these two weeks are a great time to reduce the amount of caffeine from your system. Limit the amount to 1-2 cups (8-16 oz) and only in the morning. If you struggle with decreasing your caffeine consumption or crave the taste in the afternoon, try Teeccino herbal coffee alternative, www.teeccino.com. No artificial sweeteners at all though! If you have to use a sweetener make it a teaspoon of raw honey or a touch of stevia. Again though, this is now a sugary beverage and you risk storing excess weight. Herbal tea is acceptable. Just don't let drinking coffee or tea interfere with drinking enough water throughout the day.

It's probably no surprise that my recommended drink of choice is filtered water at room temperature. If you just can't stand the taste of water try adding slices of lemon, cucumber, oranges, etc. to change the flavor. You'll be surprised; once your body begins to get fully hydrated you will actually crave water.

In order to figure how much water you should drink, take your current weight and divide by two. That is the number of ounces of water you should drink each day. Add more for exercising or warm climates. If you haven't been drinking water, don't jump to your goal right away. Add 6-8 ounces of additional water every other day until you reach your goal. Don't forget to redo your math as your weight decreases!

When you drink liquids is just as important as which ones you choose. Your body can only metabolize about 4 ounces of water every 15 minutes, so downing 32 ounces all at once to get caught up on your goal is just going to make you visit the restroom frequently. Sip on water throughout the day. Try to refrain from drinking much while eating to keep from diluting digestive juices.

Start with a big glass of water when you wake up. If you are having difficulty being hungry within the 30 minutes for breakfast, add 1-2 Tbs. of apple cider vinegar to the water first thing in the morning. This will get your digestive juices flowing. You can also drink a cup of water with 1-2 Tbs. apple cider vinegar about 30 minutes before lunch and dinner to help with digestion.

# MEAL PLAN BASICS AND HELPFUL HINTS

The 2 Week Weight Loss Program isn't difficult to follow. Each meal and snack is listed and recipes are provided with a complete grocery list for each week. Healthy tips are offered whenever possible to speed up the process, make you more efficient, or help you find the healthiest choices.

Remember to space your meals and snacks for every few hours depending on the number of hours you will be awake. Don't eat later than two hours prior to bed so your food will be mostly digested before sleeping.

Some recipes designate food as organic while others don't specify. If it is within your finances to purchase organic foods it will be in your best health interest as well as the best interest of the environment overall. If you have to pick and choose how you are spending at the grocery store, focus on meats and fats first as well as spinach and strawberries. Each species of animal, including human, makes its own characteristic kinds of triglycerides, which is governed by genetics. But, fats in the diet can affect the types of triglycerides made. As an example, animals raised for food can be fed diets containing softer or harder triglycerides to give the animal softer or harder fat, depending on consumer demand. This is why it's so important to eat organic, pasture raised meats rather than factory farmed meats. Spinach and strawberries have been proven to be highly absorbent of pesticides, which our bodies identify as toxins. All toxins are stored in fat; extra toxins require additional fat storage which may increase your overall weight. In other words, your body will make additional fat and weight to store toxins in order to keep toxins away from vital organs. In order to reduce weight you have to reduce toxin ingestion.

Each year the Environmental Working Group compares conventionally grown fruits and vegetables to identify the 12 with the most and least pesticide, herbicide, and insecticide residue. You can reduce your toxin load by following this list. You can find more information about detoxification in my book Cleanse and Detoxify You Body: 28 days to better health using nutrient-dense whole foods.

Breakfast and lunch recipes are one serving unless you will be saving extra servings for future meals/snacks. To make the best use of your time and energy, leftovers will be used. Dinner recipes are four servings with an occasional leftover used to make a later meal/snack. Remember to adjust the serving size to fit your household.

Vegetable broth is frequently used. If you have time to make your own stock, fabulous! But, if you are too busy, boxed broth is acceptable. I have recommended vegetable broth because it is currently the most common

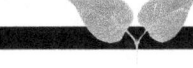

broth that doesn't have added sweeteners. If you have a chicken or beef broth you love that doesn't have added sweetener, by all means use it and let me know the name.

It is recommended to make your own aioli (mayonnaise) and a recipe is included. Making your own ensures the best quality ingredients with no added sugars. If you don't have the time then purchase Hain Safflower Mayonnaise.

If you find a new food or a food you haven't liked in the past on the menu, I recommend you give it a try. Tastes change. How food is prepared makes a difference. Don't discount it until you've tried it. Tried it and hate it? Go ahead and substitute one of the other recipes – just don't substitute lunches and dinners for snacks.

At no point in the 2 Week Weight Loss Program should you be overly hungry. Each meal includes lots of vegetables but if you are still hungry, add additional vegetables. There is really no limit to the amount of vegetables you eat as long as they were in the recipe (i.e. no adding potatoes to roasted vegetables). Don't add extra protein as your body can only process a certain amount of protein at a given time; extra will lead to weight gain.

Don't skip meals or snacks. If you're not hungry, eat a few bites to keep your metabolism revved. You won't lose weight by skipping meals. When the body is deprived of nutrients it will begin to store fat and weight for fear of a famine situation (most of us in first world countries don't live in famine situations anymore but the body is still designed to combat this potential catastrophe).

If you're not a sweets person and don't want to eat the dessert, that's fine. It's a nice treat for those of us who have sweet tooths and can help make the two weeks more endurable. I recommend Love Bean Essentially Raw Superfood Fudge Spread for a little chocolate hit that many need. Find it at Amazon.

Most of all, keep your eye on the prize – your goal is to look fabulous quickly!

## LEA'S STORY – Less Pain Now

*Lea had a lot of aches and pains when we first met. Not understanding the role of fat in our bodies she had been on a low fat, calorie counting diet most of her life. Unfortunately this had led to severe nutrient deficiencies. "I thought I was eating all the right foods: the low fat low calorie and what I thought was balanced meals. Was I wrong. Kellie has set me on the right path to proper nutrition and eating the right food. I've learned so much from Kellie and The Right Plan!" Now Lea is careful to add a good quality fat to her meals. Her body is emulsifying and utilizing these fats to decrease her level of pain. She is regularly working out, something she hadn't been able to do in years, while easily maintaining a proper weight.*

# PLANNING AND PREPARATION TIPS

Adjusting to spending time in the kitchen can be overwhelming for some people, but it doesn't have to be. Start by planning. With this book, you have the menu already laid out. You have the grocery list prepared. Items are grouped together for easier, faster shopping. Check which items you already have on hand and cross them out. I recommend rewriting the list assembling the necessary items together based on the layout of your market so you don't have to walk back and forth across the store. You may have to visit a grocery store and a health food store depending on your area. If there are items you can't find, check the internet and get them ordered.

Plan a little extra time to shop, especially if you will be looking for items you haven't purchased before. If you have the ability to purchase fresh fish the day you will be eating it, this is the best. Plan to prep as many items in advance as possible. Chop vegetables for salads, cook turkey or chicken breasts, make dressings, wash lettuce leaves, etc. Time spent one day will save you lots of time later and reduce your stress. Put on your favorite music and enjoy a couple hours spent knowing you are losing weight while prioritizing your health; visualize the new you after the 2 Week Weight Loss Program.

Each day lists "make ahead" items. Check these every night after dinner or before bed. Having these ready to go will save you frustration, eating too late, skipping foods, or ordering pizza because you weren't prepared.

Planning ahead is the best indicator of success with the 2 Week Weight Loss Program!

## CHANDRA'S STORY – Planning Isn't That Tough & I'm Down 80 lbs!

*Chandra never bothered to plan ahead for her meals. Soon she was stopping frequently at fast food restaurants and gaining weight. Although a wonderful cook, she only cooked when she felt she had time. "I didn't realize how a little planning and a little prep work made cooking quick and easy. Every Sunday part of our family routine is to map out our meals, grocery shop, and prepare for the week. It's actually simple and fun." Chandra has lost weight every week since she started planning her meals and saved enough money to take their first family vacation. Currently she's lost more than 80 pounds! "My son loves these recipes. I couldn't get him to eat vegetables until I started using Kellie's recipes."*

# WHAT DOES PROPERLY SOAKED MEAN?

Many of the recipes call for properly soaked beans. This is important to your overall health and will improve your digestive system. All beans, nuts, seeds and grains contain acids, sugars, or starches useful for germination as protection until the bacteria in the ground eat the exterior allowing sprouting. Untreated this can combine with calcium, magnesium, copper, iron and especially zinc in the intestinal tract and block their absorption or cause digestive distress in humans though.

Soaking allows enzymes, lactobacilli, and other helpful organisms to break down and neutralize the food. Soaking will neutralize a large portion. Soaking also neutralizes enzyme inhibitors and encourages the production of numerous beneficial enzymes. The action of these enzymes also increases the amounts of many vitamins, especially B vitamins which provide extra energy.

In the 2 Week Weight Loss Program grains will not be used. Since soaking is new to most people I've limited it to just the beans in this program. If you have the time and desire, soaking nuts and seeds is a tremendous health advantage. I'm including steps for both. In some of the recipes I have given an option to use canned beans. This is not ideal but I understand soaking may be more than you have time to undertake during the 2 Week Weight Loss Program.

If you choose to purchase canned beans make sure the can states BPA-free. Bisphenol-A (BPA) is a known endocrine disruptor causing negative health effects. Many people are aware of the danger of BPA in plastic but are unaware that canned goods use BPA liners.

**Soaking Beans:** cover beans with warm water. For black beans and lentils add 1 Tbs. whey or lemon juice for each cup of water. Leave in a warm place for 12-24 hours depending on the size of the bean. Lentils only soak for 7 hours. Drain, rinse, place in a large pot, and cover beans with water. Bring to a boil and skim off foam. Reduce heat, simmer covered for 4-8 hours (until tender) adding more water as necessary. Lentils only cook for about an hour.

**Soaking Nuts:** place in bowl, fill with water, you can add sea salt if you'd like, let sit for about 12 hours. Some people like them just like this, others like to dry them back out by placing them on a cookie sheet in the oven at your lowest possible temperature. In my house it takes about another 12 hours to get them to the crunchy state the family likes. Let your taste be your guide though.

# WHAT HAPPENS AFTER THE TWO WEEKS?

The 2 Week Weight Loss Program is designed to provide the jump start you need and ensure you look and feel your best. It will detoxify your body from some of the most potential allergens and balance your system. You will have more energy, think clearer, feel better, and lose weight. For most people though it's not realistic to have this be a permanent way of life – we all have dinners out, holidays, food related meetings, etc. In order to continue along a path toward optimal health and weight loss you will have to cook most of your foods though. Luckily, by the end of the two weeks you will have a pretty good idea of how cooking can fit within your schedule even if it's at a less intense commitment.

The basics of the 2 Week Weight Loss Program are a good format for a permanent eating plan. Continue eating three meals a day and two snacks emphasizing good quality proteins and fats. Consider a protein shake in place of whole food snacks if you need to reduce your amount of time in the kitchen. Minimize the use of starchy carbohydrates and sugars. Then the occasional party food won't derail your progress; just get back to a healthy eating plan with your next meal or snack.

Nutrient dense whole foods will lead to your ideal weight and energy all day but sometimes you may need to choose a processed food. Learn how to make the best choices by understanding how to read the nutrition label, nutrition data, ingredient list, and what it all really means by listening to the Processed Foods episode of my radio show Eat Well to Live Well with Kellie Hill http://www.voiceamerica.com/episode/76362/processed-foods-the-devil-we-know-and-how-to-make-the-best-choices.

For more free recipes and continued support visit www.therightnutritionplan. com. Here you will find healthy recipes, nutrition tips, articles, blogs, forums, videos, classes and more to help you maintain your success or carry on toward your ultimate goal. You don't have to stop now that you've started!

When you're ready to continue your personal journey and create permanent change visit www.eatrightforlifeplan.com. This is a twelve module program that is the secret to my client's amazing successes. This powerful plan will teach you to eat the foods that are in the best harmony with the metabolic needs of your body. You will easily lose excess fat, have increased energy, reduced appetite, loss of cellulite, less food cravings, improved digestion, and enhanced moods. You can reach your goals easily by understanding where you get your energy, where you store fat, what types of foods you should eat, and how to reach your goals. Just like the 2 Week Weight Loss Program, this is not a fad diet, it's not a one-size-fits-all diet. The Eat Right For Life Plan is real food you purchase at your grocery store with a plan to achieve your ideal weight and have energy all day in a healthy way. You learn to make your own healthy eating plan and how to eat right for yourself - permanently. At the Eat Right for Life Live Workshop you will also learn to tweak your family favorite recipes to be healthier. You achieve your goals. Find more information about this remarkable program at www.eatrightforlifeplan.com.

## SHANNON STORY – I've Lost More Than My Goal

*Shannon struggled with her weight and nutrition her entire life. Unfortunately as a busy, successful business woman she was constantly on the go. "I really had no idea what I was putting into my body." First we eliminated some of the major potential allergens, just like in the 2 Week Weight Loss Program. Her digestion problems went away, her energy level increased, and she started to lose weight. She decided on a goal weight prior to her wedding and I introduced her to the 2 Week Weight Loss Program. Shannon was so successful that her dress had to be altered multiple times. "Using the basic principles I've lost more weight than I thought I could. My life has completely changed for the better. I look and feel fantastic!"*

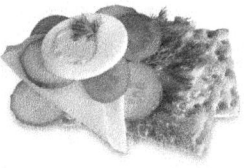

# meal plans

# SHOPPING LIST – WEEK 1

## PRODUCE

apples, 2
avocado, 1 1/4
broccoli, 1 3/4 cup
Brussels sprouts, fresh, 4 oz
butternut squash, 2 cups
carrots, 3
cauliflower, 1/4 head
celery, 2 bunches
cherry tomatoes, 1/4 pint
cilantro, fresh, 2 T
cucumber, 1
Dates, 3
dill, fresh 5 T plus a few springs
    or 3 tsp dried
garlic cloves, 29
ginger root, 3 T , approx. 3 in. piece
green onions, 2
kale, curly, 1 bunch
kale, Italian flat, 1/4 bunch
lemons, 5
limes, 3
mint, fresh, 2 T
mixed green salad mix, organic, 4 cups
mushrooms, 16
onion, 1
onion, sweet, 1
orange, 1
orange juice, fresh 6 oz, approx. 3 oranges
parsley, fresh minced 2 T or 1 tsp dried
peppers of choice, 1/4 cup
raw vegetables of choice, 1 1/4 cup
red cabbage, shredded, 3/4 cup
red onion, 1/2
red pepper, 5
romaine lettuce, 2 heads
rosemary, fresh 1/2 T or 1/2 tsp dried
sage, fresh 1/4 tsp or a pinch dried
snow peas, 1/3 cup
spinach, organic, 6 cups
strawberries, 8
Swiss chard, fresh, organic, 1/2 pound
tarragon, fresh 1/4 T or 1/4 tsp dried
thyme, fresh 4 tsp
    or 1 tsp dried
tomato, 6
vegetables, 1/2 cup for steaming
    (pg. 93 for ideas)
white wine, dry, 1 T

## DRY GOODS

almond butter, 5 T
almonds, raw 1 1/4 cup
anchovies, 1/4 oz
apple cider vinegar , 3/4 cup
balsamic vinegar, 1/3 cup
basil, fresh 2 T or 2 tsp dried
beans of choice, cooked, 1 cup
    (pg. 94 for ideas) or BPA free can
black beans, cooked 1 1/2 cups
    or 15 oz BPA free can
black pepper, fresh ground, 1/4 tsp
brown rice protein powder, 3 T
capers, 2 1/4 T
coconut aminos, 2 1/4 T
coconut milk, 1 1/4 cup
coconut oil, 9 1/2 T
coconut sugar, 1 1/2 T
corn tortillas, organic, 4
dijon mustard, 5 1/2 T
dried cranberries, 1 1/2 T
dried fruit(s) of choice, 1/2 cup total
    (pg. 60 for ideas)
extra virgin olive oil, organic, 3 cups
kalamata olives, 14
lentils, 1/4 cup cooked
    or BPA-free can
nut oil, 1 T
raisins, 1 cup
raw honey or coconut sugar, 1/4 cup
raw honey, 3 1/2 T
raw nuts of choice, 1 cup total
    (pg. 60 for ideas)
raw seeds of choice, 1/4 cup total
    (pg. 60 for ideas)
red wine vinegar, 1 1/2 T
rice vinegar, 1 T
salsa, 2 cups +
sesame oil, raw, 3/4 cup + 1/4 T
sesame seeds, 3 T
tahini, 2 1/2 T
unsweetened chocolate, 6 squares
unsweetened coconut, 1/2 T
vanilla extract, real not flavored, 1/2 tsp
vegetable broth, 2/3 cup
vegetable juice, 28 oz
walnuts, raw, 1/2 cup
Love Bean Superfudge Spread, 2 T

## PROTEIN

chicken breast, cooked, organic, 3 cups
chicken breast, organic with skin and
bone, 2
chicken breast, organic, skinless,
    boneless, 4 oz
chicken or turkey breast, organic, cooked,
    diced, 3 oz.
Italian sausage, grass fed, 1/2 pound
salmon, wild caught, 6 oz.
scallops, 5 oz.
shrimp, 3/4 lb
sirloin steak, grass fed, 4 oz
smoked salmon, thin, 8-10 slices
turkey breast, organic, sliced, 6 oz
tuna, canned, BPA-free, 2
white fish of choice, 5 oz

## DAIRY

eggs, organic, 24
parmesan, fresh grated, 1/4 tsp
white miso soup paste (refrigerated)

## FROZEN

blueberries, frozen, 1/2 cup
spinach, frozen chopped organic, 20 oz

## SPICES

cayenne, 3/4 tsp
celery salt, 1/2 tsp
chili powder, 2 tsp
crushed red pepper flakes, 1/16 tsp
cumin, ground, 3/4 tsp
curry powder, 1 tsp
fennel seeds, 1/4 tsp
sage, dried, 1/2 tsp
sea salt
white pepper, 3/4 tsp

## OPTIONAL

almonds, chopped, 2 T
avocado
baking cups
cheddar cheese, raw, shredded , 1/4 cup
cilantro, fresh, 2 T
cumin, ground, 1 tsp
flavors for kale chips (pg. 63 for ideas)
Kalamata olives, 10
macadamia nut oil, 1/4 T
paprika, 1/2 tsp
red pepper flakes

## NOTES:

The shopping list is for one person, be sure to check recipes and adjust the serving size for your household.

If you can't find an ingredient or don't want to purchase an item in order to use only a small amount, that's okay. Don't stress about ingredients. Go without a spice, switch a nut oil to olive oil, eat more of a few vegetables rather than a large variety. It's more important that you reach your weight loss goals than getting caught up in having just the right ingredients. Follow the intent of the program as close as possible and you'll still have great success.

Send me a note if you have issues, questions, or concerns—support@2weekweightlossprogram.com

# DAY 1

## Make Ahead:
*Balsamic Vinaigrette (pg. 40)*
*Red Pepper Vinaigrette (pg. 41)*
*Creamy Ginger Dressing*
*(pg. 42)*
*Red Pepper Hummus (pg. 58)*
*Aioli (pg. 43)*

## BREAKFAST:
Breakfast Scramble (pg. 47)
4 oz. Vegetable Juice

## SNACK:
1 – 2 Turkey Wraps (pg. 57)

## LUNCH:
Chicken Salad (pg. 67)
2 Tbs. Balsamic Vinaigrette

## SNACK:
Celery Sticks
1 Tbs Almond Butter

## DINNER:
4 oz. Salmon with Orange Sauce
(pg. 77)
Swiss Chard (pg. 94)
Tossed Salad (mixed greens &
chopped vegetables of choice)
2 Tbs. Red Pepper Vinaigrette

## DESSERT:
4 organic strawberries dipped in 1
Tbs. Love Bean Superfood Fudge
Spread (warmed if desired)

# DAY 2

## Make Ahead:
*Chocolate Meringue Cookies*
*(pg. 118)*
*Trail Mix (pg. 59) –*
*recommended to make 4*
*servings to last for the two*
*weeks*

## BREAKFAST:
3 Mini Quiches (save extras for
leftovers) (pg. 48)
4 oz. vegetable juice

## SNACK:
2 Tbs. Red Pepper Hummus
Raw vegetables of choice

## LUNCH:
Stuffed Tomato (pg. 68)

## SNACK:
¼ cup Trail Mix (pg. 59)

## DINNER:
3 – 4 oz. Baked Chicken Breast with
Herbs (pg. 78)
Steamed Vegetables (pg. 95)
½ cup Puréed Beans (pg. 96)

## DESSERT:
1 Almond Bar (pg. 117)

# DAY 3

**Make Ahead:**
*Shrimp Salad (pg. 70)*
*Black Bean Hummus (pg. 60)*

## BREAKFAST:
Morning Scramble (pg. 49)
4 oz. Vegetable Juice

## SNACK:
1-2 Turkey Wraps (pg. 57)

## LUNCH:
Chopped Salad (pg. 69)

## SNACK:
½ Apple
1 Tbs Almond Butter

## DINNER:
3-4 oz. Sirloin Steak (pg. 79)
Roasted Brussels Sprouts (pg. 97)
Tomato Slices with 1 Tbs. Balsamic
Vinaigrette
Mashed Butternut Squash (pg. 98)

## DESSERT:
3 Chocolate Meringue Cookies

# DAY 4

**Make Ahead:**
*Florida Rolls mixture (pg. 61)*
*Kale Chips (pg. 62)*

## BREAKFAST:
Spinach Frittata (save ½ mixture for
leftovers) (pg. 50)
4 oz. Vegetable Juice

## SNACK:
Celery Sticks
1 Tbs. Almond Butter

## LUNCH:
Shrimp Salad (pg. 70)

## SNACK:
2 Tbs. Black Bean Hummus
Raw Vegetables of Choice

## DINNER:
3 – 4 oz. Mustard Chicken (pg. 80)
Boiled Spinach (pg. 99)
Tossed Salad (mixed greens &
chopped vegetables of choice)
2 Tbs. Creamy Ginger Dressing

## DESSERT:
Blueberry Ice (pg. 119)

# DAY 5

## BREAKFAST:
Spicy Breakfast Burrito (save ½ mixture for leftovers) (pg. 51)
4 oz. Vegetable Juice

## SNACK:
Florida Rolls

## LUNCH:
Curried Chicken Salad (save ½ mixture for leftovers) (pg. 71)

## SNACK:
1 (leftover) Mini Quiche
Kale Chips

## DINNER:
4 oz. Quick Scallops (pg. 81)
Caesar Salad (pg. 100)
Red Cabbage and Snow Pea Salad (pg. 101)

## DESSERT:
Apple Treat (pg. 120)

# DAY 6

## BREAKFAST:
(leftover) Spinach Frittata
4 oz. Vegetable Juice

## SNACK:
1-2 Turkey Wraps (pg. 57)

## LUNCH:
(leftover) Shrimp Salad

## SNACK:
¼ cup Trail Mix

## DINNER:
3- 4 oz. Baked Chicken (pg. 82)
½ cup Lentils (pg. 102)
Pickled Kale Salad (pg. 103)

## DESSERT:
4 organic strawberries dipped in 1 Tbs. Love Bean Superfood Fudge Spread (warmed if desired)

# DAY 7

**Make Ahead:**
  *Florida Rolls mixture (pg. 61)*

## BREAKFAST:
3 (leftover) Mini Quiches
4 oz. Vegetable Juice

## SNACK:
Celery Sticks
1 Tbs Almond Butter

## LUNCH:
Stuffed Tomato (pg. 68)

## SNACK:
2 Tbs. Red Pepper Hummus
Raw Vegetables of Choice

## DINNER:
4 oz. Lemon Fish (pg. 83)
Mashed Cauliflower (pg. 104)
Grilled Romaine Salad (pg. 105)

## DESSERT:
1 Almond Bar

# SHOPPING LIST – WEEK 2

## PRODUCE

apple, 1
asparagus, 1 pound
avocado, 2
beet, 1 large or 2 small
bell pepper, 1
broccoli, 3 cups
butternut squash, 1 1/4 cup
carrot, 1 1/2
celery, 1 bunch
cilantro, fresh chopped, 4 1/4 T
cucumber, 1
garlic cloves 15
ginger root, minced, 1/2 T
green chilis, mild, chopped, 1/4 T
green onions, 3
jalapeno pepper, 1/4
kale, curly, one head
kale, Italian, 1/4 head
lemon , 4 1/2
lime, 1
mixed greens salad mix, 8-10 cups
mushrooms, 1/2 pound
Napa cabbage, thin sliced, 1 cup + 4
leaves
onion, 1
orange, 2
parsley, fresh, chopped 1 1/4 T or 1 1/4 tsp
dried
parsley, fresh, minced, 1/2 tsp
raw vegetables of choice, 2 cup
red onion, 1/4
red pepper, 1 1/2
romaine, 4 leaves
shallot, minced ,2 T
snow peas, 4
spinach, baby, organic, 5 cups
strawberries, 8
Swiss chard, 1/2 pound
thyme, fresh springs 2-3
tomato, 1 1/4
yellow beet, 1/4
yellow pepper, 1/4
zucchini, 1/2

## DRY GOODS

almond butter, 5T
almonds, chopped, 1 T
artichoke hearts, water packed, 1/4 jar,
approx. 2 oz.
balsamic vinegar, 2 tsp
black beans, cooked, 1 cup or BPA-free can
capers, 1/4 T
coconut aminos, 1 1/2 tsp
coconut milk, 1 cup
coconut oil, 10 1/2 T
dry red wine, 2 T
extra virgin olive oil, organic, 1/2 cup
ghee, organic, 1/4 T
honey, raw, 2 T
Kalamata olives, 9
panko 1/4 T
parchment paper
quinoa, 1/4 cup
rice vinegar, 1/2 T
salsa
sesame oil, 1/2 tsp
tomato paste, 1/4 tsp
unsweetened coconut, 1/2 T
vegetable broth, 3/4 cup
vegetable juice, 28 oz
Love Bean Superfudge Spread, 1 T
wine vinegar, 1/4 T

## PROTEIN

chicken breast, organic, cooked, 5 1/2 cups
chicken breast, organic, boneless, skinless,
1
chicken or turkey breast, cooked, diced,
3 oz.
cod, 5 oz
halibut, wild caught, 5 oz
ham, nitrate free, cooked, cubed, 4 oz
London broil, grass fed, 6 oz
smoked salmon, thin 8-10 slices
snapper, grouper, halibut, or salmon filet,
wild caught, 1/4 pound
turkey breast, organic, sliced, 2 oz.
turkey or chicken breast, cooked, cubed
4 oz

## DAIRY

eggs, organic, 9
Monterey Jack cheese, raw, 1/4 oz
parmesan cheese, fresh grated, 1/4 T
white miso soup paste (refrigerated)

## FROZEN

blueberries, frozen 1 cup
peas, frozen, 4 oz

## SPICES

bay leaf, 1
black pepper, fresh ground
cayenne, 1/2 tsp
chili powder, pinch
coriander, ground 1/4 tsp
cracked black pepper, fresh 1/4 tsp
cumin, ground 1/4 tsp
oregano, fresh chopped 1/4 T or 1/4 tsp
dried
red pepper flakes, 1/4 tsp
sea salt
thyme, dried, pinch
white pepper, 1/4 tsp

## NOTES:

The shopping list is for one person, be sure to check recipes and adjust the serving size for your household.

If you can't find an ingredient or don't want to purchase an item in order to use only a small amount, that's okay. Don't stress about ingredients. Go without a spice, switch a nut oil to olive oil, eat more of a few vegetables rather than a large variety. It's more important that you reach your weight loss goals than getting caught up in having just the right ingredients. Follow the intent of the program as close as possible and you'll still have great success.

Send me a note if you have issues, questions, or concerns – support@2weekweightlossprogram.com

# DAY 8

### Make Ahead:
*2 servings Orange Broccoli Chicken (pg. 72)*

### BREAKFAST:
(leftover) Spicy Breakfast Burrito
4 oz. Vegetable Juice

### SNACK:
Florida Rolls

### LUNCH:
(leftover) Curried Chicken Salad

### SNACK:
Kale Chips

### DINNER:
Fish in Parchment (pg. 84)
Spinach Salad (pg. 106)

### DESSERT:
Blueberry Ice (pg. 119)

# DAY 9

### BREAKFAST:
Vegetable Omelet (pg. 52)
4 oz. Vegetable Juice

### SNACK:
1-2 Turkey Wraps (pg. 57)

### LUNCH:
Orange Broccoli Chicken (save ½ mixture for leftovers) (pg. 72)

### SNACK:
1 (leftover) Mini Quiche
Kale Chips

### DINNER:
Mexican Stuffed Chicken (pg. 85)
½ cup Mexican Quinoa with Spinach (pg. 107)
Roasted Asparagus (pg. 108)

### DESSERT:
3 Chocolate Meringue Cookies

# DAY 10

**Make Ahead:**
  *Florida Rolls mixture (pg. 61)*

## BREAKFAST:
Morning Scramble (pg. 49)
4 oz. Vegetable Juice

## SNACK:
Celery Sticks
1 Tbs. Almond Butter

## LUNCH:
Chef's Salad (pg. 73)
2 Tbs. Balsamic Vinaigrette

## SNACK:
2 Tbs. Black Bean Hummus
Raw Vegetables of Choice

## DINNER:
4 oz. Baked Cod (pg. 86)
15 oz. Frozen Green Peas, heated
Kale and Fruit Salad (pg. 109)

## DESSERT:
Apple Treat (pg. 120)

# DAY 11

## BREAKFAST:
3 (leftover) Mini Quiches
4 oz. Vegetable Juice

## SNACK:
Florida Roll

## LUNCH:
Chicken Salad (pg. 67)
2 Tbs. Red Pepper Vinaigrette

## SNACK:
¼ cup Trail Mix (pg. 59)

## DINNER:
3 – 4 oz. London Broil (save 2 oz to make wraps) (pg. 87)
Sautéed Onions and Mushrooms (pg. 110)
Roasted Beets (pg. 111)
Tossed Salad (mixed greens & chopped vegetables of choice)
2 Tbs. Creamy Ginger Dressing

## DESSERT:
4 organic strawberries dipped in 1 Tbs. Love Bean Superfood Fudge Spread (warmed if desired)

# DAY 12

**Make Ahead:**
*Kale Chips (pg. 62)*

## BREAKFAST:
Huevos Rancheros (pg. 53)
4 oz. Vegetable Juice

## SNACK:
1-2 London Broil Wraps (with leftover London Broil) (same as Turkey Wraps pg. 57)

## LUNCH:
Orange Broccoli Chicken (leftover)

## SNACK:
½ Apple
1 Tbs. Almond Butter

## DINNER:
Chicken Piquant (pg. 88)
Swiss Chard (pg. 94)
Cabbage Salad (pg. 112)

## DESSERT:
1 Almond Bar

# DAY 13

**Make Ahead:**
*Florida Rolls mixture (pg. 61)*

## BREAKFAST:
Vegetable Omelet (pg. 52)
4 oz. Vegetable Juice

## SNACK:
1 (leftover) Mini Quiche
Kale Chips

## LUNCH:
Chef's Salad (pg. 73)
2 Tbs. Red Pepper Vinaigrette

## SNACK:
¼ cup Trail Mix (pg. 59)

## DINNER:
1 cup Miso Soup (white miso paste mixed with water – look for miso paste in the refrigerated section)
Cabbage Spring Rolls (pg. 89)

## DESSERT:
Blueberry Ice (pg. 119)

# DAY 14

## BREAKFAST:
Huevos Rancheros (pg. 53)
4 oz. Vegetable Juice

## SNACK:
Celery Sticks
1 Tbs. Almond Butter

## LUNCH:
Chopped Salad (pg. 69)

## SNACK:
Florida Rolls

## DINNER:
4 oz. Tangy Halibut (pg. 90)
Roasted Vegetables (pg. 113)
Tossed Salad (mixed greens &
chopped vegetables of choice)
2 Tbs. Balsamic Vinaigrette

## DESSERT:
3 Chocolate Meringue Cookies

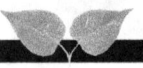

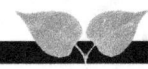

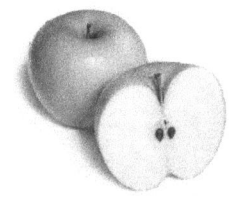

# recipes

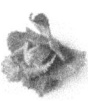

# dressings

# Balsamic Vinaigrette

## INGREDIENTS:

- ⅔ cup extra-virgin olive oil
- ⅓ cup balsamic vinegar
- 2 tsp. chopped fresh thyme or ½ tsp. dried thyme
- 1 Tbs. chopped fresh basil or 1 tsp. dried basil
- 2 cloves of garlic, pressed
- ¼ tsp. sea salt
- ⅛ tsp. white pepper

## DIRECTIONS:

Whisk all ingredients together or combine all ingredients in a jar, cover and shake.

# Red Pepper Vinaigrette

## INGREDIENTS:

- One red bell pepper, chopped
- 2 Tbs. lemon juice
- ½ cup extra virgin olive oil
- 3 cloves garlic
- Pinch cayenne
- ½ tsp. sea salt
- ⅓ cup water

## DIRECTIONS:

Mix all ingredients in a blender. Blend for one minute on high speed until creamy. Add more water as needed until desired consistency.

# Creamy Ginger Dressing

## INGREDIENTS:

- 1 Tbs. Dijon mustard
- ¼ cup apple cider vinegar
- 3 Tbs. coconut aminos
- 1 Tbs. white miso
- 1 sm.all carrot, coarsely chopped
- 1 tsp. grated ginger
- 3 pitted dates
- 2 Tbs. tahini
- ¾ cup raw sesame oil

## DIRECTIONS:

Mix all ingredients except oil in a blender. Blend for one minute on high speed until creamy. Drizzle oil into blender until dressing becomes creamy.

# Aioli (Mayonnaise)

## INGREDIENTS:

- *1 garlic clove, skinned & finely chopped*
- *2 large egg yolks*
- *1 Tbs. Dijon mustard*
- *1 cup extra virgin olive oil*
- *2 Tbs. lemon juice or white wine vinegar*
- *½ tsp. fine sea salt*
- *freshly ground white pepper*

## OPTIONAL:

*½ avocado, mashed*

*1 tsp fresh ground cumin*

*2 Tbs. chopped fresh cilantro*

*Dash spicy Hungarian paprika*

*Pinch red pepper flakes*

*Lime instead of lemon*

*Lime or lemon zest*

## DIRECTIONS:

1. Chop garlic and let sit for 5-10 minutes.
2. Combine the garlic, egg yolks, mustard, salt & pepper in a food processor. Process until well blended. Scrape down sides of bowl occasionally.
You can also use a hand whisk.
3. Very gradually add oil to egg yolks in a thin steady stream with food processor going.
4. As the sauce thickens, add lemon juice. Blend well.
5. Mix in any optional ingredients.
6. Cover and refrigerate.
7. If thinner consistency is desired, thin with cold water and/or additional lemon juice.

**HELPFUL HINT:** Aioli can be a bit tricky to make but homemade has a wonderful taste not found in a processed mayonnaise. Allow the eggs and oil warm to room temperature prior to using. The oil must be added very, very gradually in order to emulsify. Don't rush this recipe.

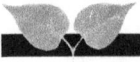

# breakfasts

# Breakfast Scramble

## INGREDIENTS:

- *1 cup red pepper, chopped*
- *½ cup onions, chopped*
- *1 cup broccoli, chopped*
- *½ cup mushrooms, sliced*
- *1 clove garlic, minced*
- *2 tsp. coconut oil*
- *2 organic eggs*
- *1 organic egg white*
- *2 Tbs. water*
- *2 Tbs. vegetable broth*
- *Salsa*

## DIRECTIONS:

1. Chop onions and garlic and allow to sit for 5-10 minutes.
2. Chop red pepper and broccoli.
3. Whisk together eggs, egg white, and water.
4. Sauté vegetables in vegetable broth until tender.
Cover and steam if necessary.
5. Add the garlic for 30 seconds.
6. Add the egg mixture and cook until desired doneness.
7. Top with salsa if desired.


**HELPFUL HINT:** Feel free to substitute other green vegetables in this recipe such as asparagus or green beans. Frozen vegetables will work also. Just place frozen vegetables in colander and run water over them until they are thawed or place in refrigerator to thaw the night before.

You can make your own salsa by adding a tomato, ¼ of a small red onion, ¼ of a jalapeno, 2 Tbs. cilantro, and 1 Tbs. lime juice in the food processor. Pulse until desired chunkiness.

**Serves 1**

# Mini Quiche

## INGREDIENTS:

- *10 oz frozen chopped organic spinach*
- *3 organic eggs*
- *3 organic egg whites*
- *2 Tbs. water*
- *¼ cup pepper, diced*
- *¼ cup sweet onion, diced*
- *Coconut oil or baking cups*

## DIRECTIONS:

1. Preheat oven to 350 degrees.
2. Place spinach in strainer. Run water over until thawed or leave in refrigerator overnight to thaw.
3. Remove excess liquid from spinach by pressing the spinach with a large spoon while still in strainer.
4. Prepare muffin pan with coconut oil.
5. Whisk eggs, egg whites, and water. Stir in other ingredients until well mixed. Divide evenly among muffin pan or cups.
6. Bake for 15-20 minutes or until a knife inserted in the center comes out clean.

**HELPFUL HINT:** Baking cups can be used with this recipe. Just be sure to coat them well with the coconut oil so the egg mixture doesn't get stuck in the creases.

If you aren't using baking cups, you can use a paper towel with a little coconut oil on it, and then run the paper towel around the muffin pan to grease. This is actually a bit healthier and more economical.

**Serves 4**

# Morning Scramble

## INGREDIENTS:

- ½ cup cooked cubed chicken
- ¼ cup peppers
- ¼ cup onions
- 1 clove garlic
- ¼ cup broccoli
- ¼ cup mushrooms
- 3 kalamata olives
- 2 Tbs. vegetable broth

## DIRECTIONS:

1. Dice onions and mince garlic. Allow to sit for 5-10 minutes.
2. Chop peppers and broccoli. Slice mushrooms. Halve olives.
3. Heat vegetable broth in skillet. Add all ingredients except garlic. Sauté until vegetables are tender but still crisp.
4. Add garlic and sauté for another minute. Serve.

**Serves 1**

# Spinach Frittata

## INGREDIENTS:

- *1 Tbs. coconut oil*
- *1 small onion, sliced*
- *2 cloves garlic, minced*
- *10 ounce package organic, frozen spinach*
- *2 organic eggs*
- *3 organic egg whites*
- *⅓ cup coconut milk*
- *¼ cup raw cheddar cheese, shredded (optional)*
- *Salsa*

## DIRECTIONS:

1. Preheat oven to 350 degrees.
2. Slice onions and mince garlic. Allow to sit for 5-10 minutes.
3. Thaw spinach by placing in strainer and running water over it until thawed. Use the back of a spoon to squeeze out most of the liquid. Or thaw in refrigerator overnight.
4. Beat eggs and egg whites with the milk until light yellow and frothy.
5. Heat oil over medium heat in a 10" skillet. Add the onion and cook, stirring, for 2 minutes. Add garlic and cook, stirring, for another minute.
6. Stir in spinach. Reduce heat to low.
7. Pour egg mixture over spinach in skillet. Cook for 5-7 minutes without stirring. Mixture should be cooked on the bottom and almost set on top.
8. Sprinkle with cheese. Bake in the oven for 5-10 minutes. Eggs should be set and cheese melted.
9. Serve topped with salsa.

**HELPFUL HINT:** Use BPA free canned coconut milk for the best consistency.

You can make your own salsa by adding a tomato, ¼ of a small red onion, ¼ of a jalapeno, 2 Tbs. cilantro, and 1 Tbs. lime juice in the food processor. Pulse until desired chunkiness.

**Serves 2**

# Spicy Breakfast Burrito

## INGREDIENTS:

- ½ cup onion
- 2 cloves of garlic
- 1 small sweet red bell pepper
- ½ pound grass fed Italian sausage
- 1 tsp coconut oil
- 3 organic eggs
- 2 organic egg whites
- 2 Tbs. water
- 2 tsp. chili powder
- ⅛ tsp. cayenne
- ¼ tsp. sea salt
- ½ tsp. black pepper
- 4 corn tortillas
- 1 cup salsa

## DIRECTIONS:

1. Dice onions and chop garlic and let sit for 5-10 minutes.
2. Dice bell peppers.
3. Whip eggs and egg whites with water.
4. Cook sausage. Move to one side of pan. Add coconut oil if needed.
5. Sauté onions and bell peppers until tender.
6. Add eggs to skillet and partially cook.
7. Add garlic, chili powder, cayenne pepper, salt and pepper to taste. Cook thoroughly.
8. Wrap ½ of mixture into each of the two tortillas.
9. Top with salsa.

**HELPFUL HINT:** You can make your own salsa by adding a tomato, ¼ of a small red onion, ¼ of a jalapeno, 2 Tbs. cilantro, and 1 Tbs. lime juice in the food processor. Pulse until desired chunkiness.

**Serves 2**

# Vegetable Omelet

## INGREDIENTS:

- *1 organic egg*
- *1 organic egg white*
- *2 Tbs. water*
- *½ Tbs. coconut oil*
- *3 stalks asparagus*
- *¼ cup mushrooms*
- *¼ cup onion*
- *¼ cup red pepper*
- *Small handful of spinach*
- *Salsa (optional)*

## DIRECTIONS:

1. Dice onions and allow to sit for 5-10 minutes.
2. Slice mushrooms, asparagus, and pepper. Chop spinach.
3. Whisk together egg, egg white, and water.
4. Heat oil in 10" skillet. Sauté onion, asparagus, pepper, and mushrooms just until beginning to be tender, approximately 2-3 minutes.
5. Pour in egg mixture.
6. Using an inverted spatula, life the edges of the mixture as it sets so the uncooked portion flows underneath the set portion.
7. When top is set, place spinach on top. Using spatula, fold omelet in half. Slide onto serving plate.
8. Top with salsa if desired.

**HELPFUL HINT:** Frozen asparagus will work also. Just place frozen vegetables in colander and run water over them until they are thawed or place in refrigerator to thaw the night before.

**Serves 1**

# Huevos Rancheros

## INGREDIENTS:

- *2 organic eggs*
- *½ cup soaked, cooked black beans or BPA-free can*
- *1 Tbs. extra virgin olive oil*
- *1 tsp. lemon juice*
- *Sea salt*
- *Fresh ground black pepper*
- *Pinch cayenne pepper*
- *¼ avocado*
- *Salsa*
- *2 Tbs. chopped cilantro*

## DIRECTIONS:

1. Chop cilantro and dice avocado.
2. Poach eggs.
3. Heat beans in a skillet. Mash if desired.
4. Remove beans from heat and mix in olive oil, lemon juice, salt, pepper and cayenne.
5. Place beans on plate, top with poached eggs, avocado, salsa, and cilantro.

**HELPFUL HINT:** Soak and cook a larger batch of beans. Measure out what you will need for the week and refrigerate. Put extra beans in the freezer. They will store for up to 6 months.

**Serves 1**

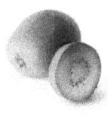

# snacks

# Turkey Wrap (& London Broil Wrap)

**INGREDIENTS:**

- *2 oz. sliced organic turkey breast*
- *4 slices red pepper*
- *½-1 Tbs. aioli*
- *Large romaine lettuce leaves*

**DIRECTIONS:**

1. Wash and dry lettuce leaves.
2. Spread aioli on lettuce leaves.
3. Add sliced turkey and red pepper.
4. Wrap/roll lettuce leaves around filling.

**HELPFUL HINT:** If you purchase deli style turkey or chicken meat make sure that it is organic, nitrate free, without hormones. Or cook a breast, slice or cube and refrigerate enough for the week. Extra meat can be frozen after cooking for up to 6 months making meals quicker and easier in the future.

**Serves 1**

# Red Pepper Hummus

## INGREDIENTS:

- *1 clove garlic*
- *2 cups soaked, cooked garbanzo beans or 1 15 oz can garbanzo beans (BPA free)*
- *2 roasted red peppers*
- *2 Tbs. lemon juice*
- *1 ½ Tbs. tahini*
- *¾ tsp. ground cumin*
- *½ tsp. salt*
- *¼ tsp. cayenne pepper*
- *¼ tsp. paprika, preferable smoked*
- *10 kalamata olives*
- *Extra virgin olive oil*

## DIRECTIONS:

1. Properly soak garbanzo beans and cook or use canned.
2. Roast red peppers or use jarred.
3. Drain and reserve liquid from garbanzo beans if using canned. Rinse.
4. Mince garlic in food processor.
5. Add beans, 2 Tbs. reserved liquid or extra virgin olive oil, and remaining ingredients. Process until smooth, scraping down the sides as needed.
6. Add additional seasonings and liquid to taste.

**Serves 8**

# Trail Mix

## INGREDIENTS:

- *Unsweetened raisins*
- *Unsweetened currants*
- *Unsweetened dried cranberries*
- *Unsweetened dried pineapple*
- *Unsweetened dried berries*
- *Unsweetened dried peaches*
- *Unsweetened dried apricots*
- *Unsweetened dried cherries*
- *Unsweetened banana chips*
- *Raw almonds*
- *Raw walnuts*
- *Raw cashews*
- *Raw pecans*
- *Raw hazelnuts*
- *Raw pistachios*
- *Raw pine nuts*
- *Raw sunflower seeds*
- *Raw pumpkin seeds*
- *Raw hemp seeds*
- *Raw chia seeds*
- *Pomegranate seeds*
- *Unsweetened coconut*

## DIRECTIONS:

1. Choose ½ cup dried fruits for each 1 cup of nuts.
2. Add ¼ cup seeds of choice.
3. 2 Tbs. coconut if desired.
4. Mix well.

# Black Bean Hummus

## INGREDIENTS:

- *1 clove garlic*
- *1 ½ cup soaked, cooked black beans or 15 oz. BPA free can*
- *2 Tbs. lemon juice*
- *1 ½ Tbs. tahini*
- *¾ tsp. ground cumin*
- *½ tsp. salt*
- *¼ tsp. cayenne pepper*
- *¼ tsp. paprika (optional)*
- *10 kalamata olives (optional)*

## DIRECTIONS:

1. Drain and reserve liquid from black beans. Rinse black beans if using canned.
2. Mince garlic in food processor, allow to sit for 5-10 minutes.
3. Add black beans, reserved liquid and remaining ingredients except paprika. Process until smooth, scraping down the sides as needed.
4. Add additional seasonings and liquid to taste.

**Serves 8**

# Florida Rolls

## INGREDIENTS:

- ½ cup butternut squash, peeled and cubed
- ½ avocado
- 1 Tbs. lime juice
- 1 Tbs. extra virgin olive oil
- 2 cloves garlic, minced
- 4-5 thin slices smoked salmon

## DIRECTIONS:

1. Steam butternut squash for 10 minutes or until tender.
2. Mash together avocado and squash. Add remaining ingredients, except smoked salmon and mix well.
3. Cool in refrigerator.
4. Lay out slices of salmon. Place a few spoonfuls of the mash on the salmon. Roll the salmon up like a sushi roll.

**HELPFUL HINT:** This recipe can be made in advance and will last in the refrigerator for up to a week.

**Serves 1**

# Kale Chips

## INGREDIENTS:

- *1 bunch kale*
- *1 Tbs. extra virgin olive oil or coconut oil*
- *¼ tsp. sea salt*

## DIRECTIONS:

1. Preheat oven to 300 degrees.
2. Wash kale. Trim away stems. Coarsely chop the leaves. It should equal about 3 cups.
3. If using coconut oil, melt.
4. Toss with oil until evenly coated.
5. Spread on a baking sheet.
6. Sprinkle with sea salt.
7. Bake for 20 minutes. They should look dried out and slightly browned when done.

## FOR ADDITIONAL FLAVOR OPTIONS TRY:

- *coconut aminos*
- *cayenne*
- *powdered garlic*
- *powdered onion*
- *sesame seeds*
- *powdered cheese*
- *lemon juice*
- *chopped nuts*
- *nutritional/brewer's yeast*
- *apple cider vinegar*
- *lime juice*
- *parmesan cheese*
- *curry powder*

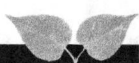

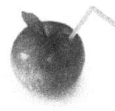

# lunches

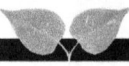

# Chicken Salad

## INGREDIENTS:

- *3 – 4 oz. organic chicken breast, sliced*
- *½ tomato, chopped*
- *½ cucumber, chopped*
- *½ carrot, chopped*
- *Additional vegetables as desired, chopped*
- *Organic spinach, approx. 2 cups but as much as you choose*

## DIRECTIONS:

1. Preheat oven to 350 degrees.
2. Pound chicken breast to ½ inch thickness. Bake for approximately 25 minutes.
3. Chop desired vegetables.
4. Wash and spin dry spinach. Place on plate.
5. Layer vegetables on spinach.
6. Top with chicken breast slices.

**Serves 1**

# Stuffed Tomato

**INGREDIENTS:**

- *1 can BPA-free or bag of tuna*
- *½ cup celery, minced*
- *1 Tbs. sweet onion, minced*
- *1 Tbs. red onion, minced*
- *1 Tbs. capers with juice*
- *1 Tbs. Dijon mustard*
- *2 Tbs. fresh dill, chopped or 1 tsp. dried dill*
- *¼ tsp. celery salt*
- *1 large tomato*

**DIRECTIONS:**

1. Mix all ingredients except tomato in a bowl.
2. Slice tomato in half, remove seeds and pulp.
3. Stuff tuna mixture into tomato halves.

**HELPFUL HINT:** This recipe can also be served over a bed of mixed greens if more food is needed. Place greens on plate, quarter tomato to top greens, add tuna mixture to middle of greens.

**Serves 1**

# Chopped Salad

**INGREDIENTS:**
- ½ cup broccoli florets
- ½ medium carrot
- 1 stalk celery
- 1 green onions
- 3 mushrooms
- ¼ medium avocado, diced
- 6 kalamata olives, pitted and chopped
- ½ tomato, diced
- 3 oz. organic chicken or turkey breast, diced

**DRESSING:**
- 1 Tbs. extra virgin olive oil
- 1 tsp. lemon juice
- 1 medium cloves garlic, pressed
- Sea salt
- White pepper

**DIRECTIONS:**
1. Press garlic and allow to sit for 5-10 minutes.
2. Mince broccoli, carrot, celery, mushrooms, and green onions using a knife or food processor. Place in a large salad bowl.
3. Add diced tomato, avocado and olives.
4. Toss with dressing until well blended.

**Serves 1**

# Shrimp Salad

## INGREDIENTS:

- ¾ lbs shrimp, peeled and deveined
- ½ head romaine lettuce or mixed greens
- 2 tomatoes, cut into wedges
- 6 fresh mushrooms, sliced
- Fresh dill sprigs, optional

## DRESSING:

- 1 ½ Tbs. extra virgin olive oil
- 1 ½ Tbs. red wine vinegar
- 1 Tbs. water
- 1 Tbs. fresh basil, chopped or 1 tsp dried basil
- 1 Tbs. fresh dill, chopped or 1 tsp dried dill
- ½ tsp garlic, pressed
- ½ tsp Dijon mustard
- ½ small onion, sliced

## DIRECTIONS:

1. Press garlic and slice onions and let sit for 5 minutes.
2. Bring small pan of water to boil over high heat. Add shrimp and cook for 3-4 minutes or until shrimp are pink and no longer translucent in the center. Drain.
3. Whisk together oil, vinegar, water, basil, dill, garlic, mustard, and onion.
4. Toss shrimp and dressing. Cover and refrigerate overnight.
5. Put lettuce on plate, add tomato wedges and mushroom slices. Top with shrimp.

**Serves 2**

# Curried Chicken Salad

## INGREDIENTS:

- *2 cups cooked organic chicken breast, cubed*
- *½ cup celery, finely chopped*
- *1 cup apples, chopped*
- *1 tsp. freshly grated ginger*
- *1 tsp. curry powder*
- *⅛ tsp. cayenne pepper*
- *¼ cup aioli*
- *1 ½ Tbs. dried cranberries*
- *One large orange to create ½ Tbs. orange zest and 2 Tbs. fresh orange juice*
- *2 cups mixed baby greens*

## DIRECTIONS:

1. Zest orange rind and juice orange.
2. In a large bowl combine all ingredients except the greens. Toss well, cover, and chill for 15 min.
3. Divide chicken salad in half, place each serving on top of mixed greens.

**Serves 2**

# Orange Broccoli Chicken

## INGREDIENTS:

- *One large bunch of broccoli florets*
- *3 Tbs. coconut oil*
- *2 cloves minced garlic*
- *1 Tbs. minced shallot*
- *Peeled rind of one orange, chopped (no white pith)*
- *⅛ tsp. red pepper flakes*
- *⅓ cup orange juice*
- *1 tsp. balsamic vinegar*
- *¼ tsp. sea salt*
- *¼ tsp. sesame oil*
- *2 cups cooked organic chicken, cubed*

## DIRECTIONS:

1. Chop broccoli florets into fairly uniform pieces. Juice orange and then chop outside of rind.
2. Sauté garlic, shallot, orange rind, and pepper flakes in coconut oil over medium heat until garlic and shallots have softened, stirring frequently.
3. Add broccoli to pan. Cook and stir 1 min.
4. Add orange juice, vinegar, salt, and chicken. Cover and steam 3 to 4 minutes over medium-high heat until broccoli is tender but still crisp.
5. Drizzle with sesame oil. Toss and serve hot or cold.

**HELPFUL HINT:** This recipe is delicious hot or cold. When preparing cold, make broccoli ahead and add chicken chunks before serving.

**Serves 1**

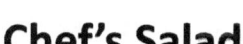

# Chef's Salad

## INGREDIENTS:

- 2 oz. cubed nitrate free ham
- 2 oz. cubed organic turkey or chicken breast
- 2-4 cups mixed greens
- Chopped vegetables of choice

## DIRECTIONS:

1. Place greens on plate.
2. Top with vegetables of choice and meats.

**Serves 1**

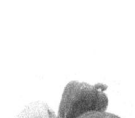

# dinners

# Salmon in Orange Sauce

## INGREDIENTS:

- 1-½ lbs wild caught salmon, cut into 4 pieces
- ½ medium sized onion, chopped
- 2 medium cloves garlic, chopped
- 2 Tbs. + 2 tsp fresh lemon juice
- 1-½ cups fresh orange juice
- 1 tsp fennel seeds
- 2 Tbs. minced fresh parsley or 2 tsp. dried parsley
- Sea salt
- White pepper

## DIRECTIONS:

1. Preheat oven to 350 degrees.
2. Chop onions and garlic, let sit for 5 minutes.
3. Season salmon pieces with 2 tsp lemon juice, salt and pepper. Bake for approximately 25 minutes or until salmon flakes easily with a fork.
4. In a small pan combine onion, garlic, fennel seeds, 2 Tbs. lemon juice, and orange juice. Cook on medium high heat until reduced in half.
5. Strain sauce over salmon to serve.
6. Sprinkle with parsley.

**Serves 4**

# Baked Chicken Breast with Herbs

## INGREDIENTS:

- *4 organic chicken breasts with skin and bones*
- *2 medium cloves garlic, pressed*
- *1 Tbs. fresh lemon juice*
- *2 tsp. chopped fresh sage or ½ tsp. dried sage*
- *2 tsp. chopped fresh thyme or ½ tsp. dried thyme*
- *2 tsp. chopped fresh rosemary or ½ tsp. dried rosemary*
- *¼ cup vegetable broth*
- *Sea salt*
- *Fresh ground black pepper*

## DIRECTIONS:

1. Preheat oven to 350 degrees.
2. Press garlic and allow to sit for 5-10 minutes.
3. Season chicken with a little salt and pepper. Bake for 25-30 minutes until chicken is no longer pink inside.
4. In a small skillet add herbs, lemon juice, broth, garlic, salt, and pepper. Heat on medium heat for about 30 seconds.
5. When chicken is done remove skin. Drizzle herb sauce over chicken.

**Serves 4**

# Sirloin Steak

## INGREDIENTS:

- *1 lb grass fed top sirloin steak*
- *Sea salt*
- *Fresh ground black pepper*
- *1 Tbs. coconut oil*

## DIRECTIONS:

1. Heat oven to 450 degrees.
2. Heat oven proof skillet over medium high until very hot. Add coconut oil. Stir until melted.
3. Add steak. Cook for 4 minutes.
4. Turn. Cook for 3-4 minutes.
5. Place skillet in oven for 3-5 minutes until desired doneness.
6. Place steak on plate, cover loosely with foil and allow to sit for 5 minutes.

**Serves 4**

# Mustard Chicken

## INGREDIENTS:

- *2 organic boneless, skinless chicken breasts, cut into 1-inch pieces*
- *1 Tbs. coconut oil*
- *1 medium onion, sliced*
- *5 medium cloves garlic, pressed*
- *3 Tbs. Dijon mustard*
- *¼ cup vegetable broth*
- *¼ cup dry white wine*
- *2 tsp raw honey*
- *1 Tbs. chopped fresh tarragon or 1 tsp. dried tarragon*
- *2 Tbs. chopped fresh parsley or 2 tsp. dried parsley*
- *Sea salt*
- *White pepper*

## DIRECTIONS:

1. Slice onion and press garlic and let sit for 5-10 minutes.
2. Cut chicken breasts into 1 inch pieces.
3. Heat coconut oil in skillet. Sauté onion until translucent.
4. Add chicken pieces and continue to sauté for another 3 minutes, stirring frequently.
5. Add garlic and continue to sauté for another minute.
6. Add mustard, broth, wine, and honey. Mix thoroughly and simmer uncovered for about 7-8 minutes on medium high heat. Stir occasionally.
7. Add seasonings. Mix and serve.

**Serves 4**

# Quick Scallops

## INGREDIENTS:

- *1 ¼ pound scallops*
- *2-4 Tbs. vegetable broth*
- *2 cloves garlic, pressed*
- *2 Tbs. extra virgin olive oil*
- *2 Tbs. lemon juice*
- *Sea salt*
- *White pepper*

## DIRECTIONS:

1. Press garlic and let sit for 5-10 minutes.
2. Whisk together oil, lemon juice, salt and pepper.
3. Heat broth in skillet until steaming.
4. Add scallops and sauté for 3-4 minutes, stirring continuously. Add additional broth to keep from burning.
5. Add garlic and continue to sauté for another minute. Remove from heat and toss with whisked ingredients. Serve.

**HELPFUL HINT:** You can use either larger scallops or small bay scallops. If using the larger scallops cut in half or quarters to make small bites. Careful not to overcook scallops as they will become tough.

**Serves 4**

# Baked Chicken

## INGREDIENTS:

- *4 organic chicken breasts, skin and bones included*
- *Sea salt*
- *Fresh ground black pepper*
- *3 Tbs. lemon juice*
- *2 cloves garlic*
- *1 ½ Tbs. chopped fresh rosemary or 2 tsp. dried rosemary*
- *1 Tbs. extra virgin olive oil*

## DIRECTIONS:

1 Preheat oven to 350 degrees.

2. Sprinkle chicken with salt and pepper.

3. Cook for 25-30 minutes or until no longer pink inside.

4. Press garlic and allow to sit for 5-10 minutes.

5. Add lemon juice, garlic, rosemary, additional salt and pepper (to taste) in small sauté pan and heat for approximately one minute.

6. Remove from heat and whisk in oil.

7. Remove skin from chicken. Drizzle sauce over chicken. Serve.

**Serves 4**

# Lemon Fish

## INGREDIENTS:

- 1 Tbs. coconut oil
- 1 ¼ lbs thin white fish (sole, tilapia, orange roughy)
- Sea salt
- Fresh ground black pepper
- 2 Tbs. macadamia nut oil or coconut oil
- 1 large clove of garlic
- 1 ½ large lemons
- 2 pints whole cherry tomatoes
- ½ cup whole pitted Kalamata or green olives
- 2 Tbs. capers
- ¼ cup chopped parsley

## DIRECTIONS:

1. Slice garlic. Allow to sit for 5-10 minutes.
2. Peal and remove pith of one lemon. Roughly chop and remove seeds.
3. Heat coconut oil in large skillet over medium high heat.
4. Evenly season the fish to taste with salt and pepper. Place in skillet and cook, undisturbed for 3-4 minutes (about ¾ cooked through). Gently flip the fish and sear the other side for 1-2 minutes, or until just cooked through.
5. As the fish cooks, heat macadamia oil in large sauté pan over medium to medium high heat. Add the lemon, and tomatoes. Sauté for 3-4 minutes until tomatoes start to soften.
6. Add the garlic, olives and capers. Sauté for 2 minutes, bursting some of the cherry tomatoes.
7. Make a bed of the lemon mixture. Arrange fish on top. Juice ½ lemon over all and garnish with parsley.

**Serves 4**

# Fish in Parchment

## INGREDIENTS:

- *1 lb snapper, grouper, halibut or salmon fillets (tail pieces)*
- *16 snow peas, strings removed, sliced on diagonal*
- *1 red pepper, julienned*
- *½ carrot, julienned*
- *2-3 cucumbers, julienned*
- *1 bunch green onions, diced*
- *4 pieces parchment paper*
- *Salt and freshly ground black pepper*
- *1 whole lemon, quartered and seeds removed*

## DIRECTIONS:

1. Preheat oven to 500 degrees.
2. Julienne cucumbers on mandolin. Sprinkle lightly with salt and let set for 15-20 minutes.
3. Slice fish at angle and pull out any bones.
4. Rinse cucumbers and drain. Pat dry.
5. In the center of one of the pieces of parchment paper, place a thin strip of julienned cucumbers. Place fish fillets on top. Next, layer red pepper strips, snow peas, carrots, and green onions on top of fish.
6. Take one quarter of the lemon and squeeze juice over fish. with salt and freshly ground pepper.
7. Bring ends of parchment paper together and roll fold middle down towards fish. Fold ends up (like a package) and then fold under the whole parchment.
8. Place fish bundles on ungreased cookie sheet. Cook for approximately 10 minutes.

**HELPFUL HINT:** You can serve this recipe in the parchment by placing the bundle on the place, unwrap or cut the top of the parchment to expose the fish and vegetables inside.

**Serves 4**

# Mexican Stuffed Chicken

## INGREDIENTS:

- *2 organic boneless, skinless chicken breasts*
- *1 tablespoon panko*
- *1 tablespoon grated Parmesan cheese*
- *2 tablespoons mild green chilis, chopped*
- *½ teaspoon chili powder*
- *1 egg, beaten*
- *1 ounce raw Monterey Jack cheese cut into two chunks*

## DIRECTIONS:

1. Preheat oven to 375 degrees.
2. With a mallet pound breasts to ¼-inch thick.
3. On each one place a tablespoon of the chilis and a Monterey Jack cheese slice.
4. Roll up and place, seam side down in a baking dish.
5. Brush with beaten egg.
6. Mix together panko, parmesan cheese and chili powder. Sprinkle over the chicken rolls, patting into place to form a crust.
7. Bake for about 20 minutes or until cooked through and crust is brown.

**HELPFUL HINT:** Make sure the chicken completely surrounds the Monterey Jack or as it melts it will ooze out and make a mess.

**Serves 4**

# Baked Cod

## INGREDIENTS:

- *1 ½ pound cod*
- *One lemon to juice plus 3 Tbs. finely grated lemon rind*
- *2 Tbs. chopped fresh parsley or 2 tsp. dried parsley*
- *¼ tsp. sea salt*
- *¼ tsp. white pepper*
- *Pinch of cayenne*

## DIRECTIONS:

1. Preheat oven to 400 degrees.
2. Chop garlic and let sit for 5-10 minutes.
3. Grate lemon rind and then juice lemon.
4. Mix together lemon rind, lemon juice, parsley, salt, pepper and cayenne.
5. Cut cod into four equal pieces. Rub generously with mixture.
6. Bake fish for 15-20 minutes or until fish flakes easily with a fork.
7. Place cod on plates. Drizzle any remaining juices from pan over fish.

**HELPFUL HINT:** Any firm white fish can be used in this recipe. Frozen is also acceptable but may take a bit longer to cook.

**Serves 4**

# London Broil

## INGREDIENTS:

- *1 ½ pound grass fed London Broil*
- *2 Tbs. extra virgin olive oil*
- *½ cup dry red wine*
- *3 cloves garlic*
- *3 Tbs. minced fresh parsley or 3 tsp. dried parsley*
- *1 Tbs. chopped fresh oregano or 1 tsp. dried oregano*
- *1 bay leaf*
- *1 tsp. fresh cracked black pepper*

## DIRECTIONS:

1. Mince garlic and allow to sit for 5-10 minutes.
2. Whisk together all ingredients except meat in a bowl or bread pan.
3. Add meat to mixture. Turn to coat ensuring all meat is covered with marinade. Cover and refrigerate overnight.
4. Preheat broiler.
5. Broil meat about 5 minutes on each side. Cover with foil and allow to sit for 5 minutes.
6. Cut into thin diagonal slices across the grain.

**Serves 4**

# Chicken Piquant

## INGREDIENTS:

- *2 organic boneless, skinless chicken breast*
- *1 tsp. coconut oil*
- *1 clove garlic, chopped*
- *1 ripe tomato, coarsely chopped*
- *1 small jar water packed artichoke hearts*
- *1 tsp. tomato paste*
- *1 Tbs. wine vinegar*
- *¼ tsp. sea salt*
- *½ tsp. dried thyme*

## DIRECTIONS:

1. Chop garlic and allow to sit 5 minutes.
2. Using a mallet, pound chicken to uniform thickness.
3. Sprinkle the chicken breast lightly with salt. Heat the oil in a frying pan and brown the chicken, about 2 minutes on each side.
4. Remove from pan and add all the remaining ingredients except the artichoke hearts.
5. Stir and heat to boiling.
6. Return the chicken to the pan, cover and cook over low heat 20-25 minutes or until chicken is tender.
7. Add the artichoke hearts for the last 5 minutes and allow to heat through.

**Serves 4**

# Cabbage Spring Rolls

## INGREDIENTS:

- *1 pound cooked shredded organic chicken*
- *Napa Cabbage leaves*
- *4 Tbs. almond butter*
- *4 tsp. honey or maple syrup*
- *4 tsp. coconut aminos*
- *4 tsp. lemon juice*
- *Dash of cayenne*
- *Shredded or thinly sliced vegetables such as carrots, zucchini, cucumbers, avocado, mushrooms.*

## DIRECTIONS:

1. Boil, roast, bake, or slow cook chicken. Using two forks shred.
2. Combine almond butter, honey, coconut aminos, lemon juice, and cayenne in small bowl.
3. Clean and trim large Napa cabbage leaves.
4. Place all items on table.
5. Spread sauce mixture on leaves. Add vegetables and chicken.
6. Roll as a wrap.

**Serves 4**

# Tangy Halibut

## INGREDIENTS:

- *1 ½ lb fresh halibut*
- *2 Tbs. coconut oil*
- *Juice of one lemon*
- *Sea salt*
- *Fresh ground pepper*
- *2-3 sprigs fresh thyme*
- *2 cloves garlic*
- *1 Tbs. capers*

## DIRECTIONS:

1. Preheat oven to 450 degrees.
2. Peel and crush garlic cloves and allow to sit for 5-10 minutes.
3. Pat the halibut dry and cut into four pieces.
4. Rub a little lemon juice on halibut, sprinkle with sea salt and fresh ground pepper.
5. Heat skillet until drop of water sizzles. Add coconut oil.
6. Sear halibut, about a minute on each side.
7. Add thyme and garlic cloves. Place skillet in oven until halibut is cooked through and fish flakes easily with fork, about 4 minutes.
8. Add remaining lemon juice and capers to pan and swirl to infuse flavors.
9. Place halibut on plates. Drizzle remaining pan dripping sauce over plate. If there isn't enough sauce left, add a little olive oil and swirl around pan.

**HELPFUL HINT:** Any firm, meaty white fish will work for this recipe. Frozen can be used as well but lower oven heat to 350 degrees and bake for 20-25 minutes or until cooked through and fish flakes easily with fork.

**Serves 4**

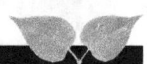

# side dishes

# Swiss Chard

## INGREDIENTS:

- *1 pound fresh Swiss chard*
- *1 tsp lemon juice (optional)*
- *2 Tbs. extra virgin olive oil*
- *Sea salt*
- *Fresh ground black pepper*

## DIRECTIONS:

1. Bring lightly salted water to a rapid boil in a large pot.
2. Wash Swiss chard. Cut off tough, bottom part of stem. If using white stems cut into ½" slices. If using red chard, remove stems and only use leaves. Cut leaves into 1" slices.
3. Place Swiss chard in boiling water. Cook uncovered for 3 minutes.
4. Drain and press out excess water in colander.
5. Toss in remaining of ingredients immediately.

**HELPFUL HINT:** It's preferable to purchase organic if possible as non-organic leafy greens have a high pesticide residue but it's not as critical as spinach, so let your finances determine your choice.

**Serves 2**

# Steamed Vegetables

## INGREDIENTS:

- *Any variety of vegetables:*
- *Carrots, sliced*
- *Onions, thick slices*
- *Squash, cubed*
- *Zucchini, cubed*
- *Broccoli, chopped*
- *Kale, chopped*
- *Celery, chopped*
- *Pepper, chopped*

## DRESSING:

- *Extra virgin olive oil*
- *Garlic, pressed*
- *Fresh lemon juice*
- *Coconut aminos*
- *Fresh chopped or dried rosemary*
- *Fresh chopped or dried thyme*
- *Sea salt*
- *Fresh ground black pepper*

## DIRECTIONS:

1. Chop onion and garlic. Allow to sit for 5-10 minutes.
2. Chop desired vegetables. Try to have uniform sizes so all vegetables are finished cooking about the same time.
3. Place vegetables in steamer. Steam for 5-8 minutes until tender but still crunchy.
4. Whisk together dressing ingredients depending on taste.
5. Remove vegetables from steamer and toss with dressing.

**Serves 4**

# Puréed Beans

**INGREDIENTS:**

- *4 cups soaked, cooked beans (cannellini, Great Northern, navy, calypso, Boston, European soldier, flageolet, marrow, mortgage runner, haricot, Steuben yellow bean, tepary, vallarta)*
- *1 medium onion, chopped*
- *4 medium cloves garlic, chopped*
- *2 tsp. coconut oil*
- *1 tsp. chopped rosemary or ¼ tsp. dried rosemary*
- *2 Tbs. vegetable broth*
- *Sea salt*
- *Fresh ground black pepper*

**DIRECTIONS:**

1. Chop onions and garlic and allow to sit for 5-10 minutes.
2. Sauté onions in oil, stirring frequently until translucent, about 5 minutes. Add garlic and continue to sauté for another minute stirring constantly.
3. Add beans, rosemary and broth. Cook for another 5 minutes or until heated through.
4. Place in blender and purée slowly. Stop the blender a few times to scrape down the sides.
5. Season with sea salt and pepper to taste.

**HELPFUL HINT:** Although any of the listed work well in this recipe, my personal favorite is tepary which was a staple of Native Americans in the Southwest. Other names for tepary beans include tapary bean and moth dal.

**Serves 4**

# Roasted Brussels Sprouts

## INGREDIENTS:

- *1 pound fresh Brussels Sprouts*
- *1 Tbs. coconut oil*
- *Sea salt*
- *Fresh black pepper*

## DIRECTIONS:

1. Preheat oven to 450 degrees.
2. Wash Brussels sprouts and remove any outer leaves that don't look good.
3. Cut into quarters and allow to sit for 5-10 minutes.
4. Place Brussels sprouts in a shallow baking dish, not glass. Add coconut oil.
5. Cook for 5 minutes in oven. Stir to evenly coat coconut oil.
6. Return to oven for another 10-15 minutes, until outside of Brussels sprouts are slightly browned.
7. Season with sea salt and pepper to taste.

**HELPFUL HINT:** Brussels sprouts can be purchased individually or on the stalk. Either is fine just remove from stalk before washing.

**Serves 4**

# Mashed Butternut Squash

## INGREDIENTS:

- *2 cups butternut squash, or any variety of winter squash*
- *3 Tbs. extra virgin olive oil*
- *1 tsp lemon juice*
- *2 cloves garlic, pressed*
- *2–4 tsp. fresh finely grated ginger (depending on tastes)*
- *sea salt*
- *white pepper*

## DIRECTIONS:

1. Peel and cut squash into 1-inch cubes.
2. Place in steamer. Steam for 10 minutes or until tender.
3. Press garlic and allow to sit for 5-10 minutes.
4. Transfer squash to food process or blender.
5. Add remaining ingredients.
6. Purée until smooth.

**Serves 2**

# Boiled Spinach

**INGREDIENTS:**

- *1 pound fresh organic spinach*
- *1 tsp lemon juice (optional)*
- *1 Tbs. extra virgin olive oil*
- *Sea salt*
- *Fresh ground black pepper*

**DIRECTIONS:**

1. Bring lightly salted water to a rapid boil in a large pot.
2. Remove stems and rinse spinach leaves to remove all dirt.
3. Cook spinach in boiling water for 30 seconds.
4. Drain and press out excess water.
5. Toss in remaining of ingredients immediately.

**HELPFUL HINT:** The easiest way to remove the stems is to leave the spinach bundled, cut at the twist tie and most of the stem can be discarded.

**Serves 2**

# Caesar Salad

## INGREDIENTS:

- 2 heads romaine lettuce
- ¼ cup walnuts

## DRESSING:

- 2 Tbs. tahini
- 1 2 oz jar anchovies
- 4 medium cloves garlic
- 3 Tbs. lemon juice
- 2 Tbs. balsamic vinegar
- 2 Tbs. extra virgin olive oil
- Sea salt
- Fresh ground black pepper

## DIRECTIONS:

1. Drain anchovies and rinse.
2. Remove and discard outer leaves of romaine.
3. Rinse lettuce, tear into bite size pieces, and spin dry (or pat on paper towels and then tear). Dry well.
4. Blend dressing ingredients together for 1-2 minutes.
5. Toss romaine lettuce with desired amount of dressing.
6. Top with walnuts.

**Serves 4**

# Red Cabbage and Snow Pea Salad

## INGREDIENTS:

- 1 ½ cups snow peas
- 3 cups red cabbage, shredded
- 1 cup carrots, grated
- 3 green onions, thin sliced
- ½ cup chopped fresh mint
- ½ cup chopped fresh cilantro
- Sea salt
- Fresh ground black pepper
- 4 tsp. sesame seeds for garnish

## DRESSING:

- 1 Tbs. coconut aminos
- 3 Tbs. nut oil
- 1 Tbs. sesame oil
- 3 Tbs. rice vinegar
- 1 inch grated fresh ginger
- Pinch of crushed red pepper flakes
- Juice of one lime
- Sea salt
- Fresh ground black pepper

## DIRECTIONS:

1. Toss all salad ingredients together.
2. Whisk all dressing ingredients together.
3. Add dressing and toss until well mixed.
4. Garnish with sesame seeds.

**Serves 4**

# Lentils

## INGREDIENTS:

- *2 cups cooked lentils*
- *1 medium onion*
- *3 cloves garlic*
- *1 Tbs. coconut oil*
- *1 ½ cup mushrooms*
- *½ tsp. dried thyme*
- *½ tsp. dried sage*
- *½ cup raw walnuts*
- *¼ cup vegetable broth*
- *Sea salt*
- *Fresh ground black pepper*

## DIRECTIONS:

1. Cook lentils by rinsing, covering with water and simmering for 20-30 minutes or until no longer tender.
2. Chop onions and garlic and allow to sit for 5-10 minutes.
3. Sauté onions and mushrooms in 1 Tbs. coconut oil until tender.
4. Add garlic, thyme and sage. Sauté another minute.
5. Add lentils, walnuts and broth. Heat thoroughly.
6. Put mixture in food processor or blender and purée. Scrape sides during blending to ensure consistent texture.

**HELPFUL HINT:** Make extra lentils and freeze them for up to 6 months. This will make future meals quicker and easier. No need to thaw frozen lentils for this recipe just heat thoroughly during step 5, which may take a bit longer.

**Serves 4**

# Pickled Kale Salad

## INGREDIENTS:

- 1 ¾ cup apple cider vinegar
- ⅓ cup coconut sugar
- 1 large cucumber
- ½ medium red onion
- Small bunch of kale
- 1 Tbsp extra virgin olive oil
- ½ tsp salt
- Freshly ground black pepper

## DIRECTIONS:

1. Thinly slice cucumber and red onion. Allow to sit for 5-10 minutes.
2. Chop kale.
3. Combine vinegar, ½ cup water, and coconut sugar in a bowl. Stir in cucumbers and onion. Set aside to let "pickle".
4. Whisk together ⅓ cup "pickling" liquid, oil, salt, and pepper. Toss with kale.
5. Strain cucumbers and onion. Toss with kale mixture.

**Serves 4**

# Mashed Cauliflower

## INGREDIENTS:

- *Large head of cauliflower*
- *Sea salt*
- *White pepper*
- *Coconut milk*

## DIRECTIONS:

1. Chop head of cauliflower.
2. Steam for 10-15 minutes or until tender.
3. Purée using pulse mode in food processor (or use potato masher) until smooth.
4. Season with salt and pepper.
5. If creamier texture is needed, add a touch of coconut milk and continue purée. Continue adding coconut milk and puréeing until desired texture is created.

**HELPFUL HINT:** Use BPA free canned coconut milk for the best consistency. Purée carefully as cauliflower can become a liquid quickly.

**Serves 4**

# Grilled Romaine

## INGREDIENTS:

- *2 heads romaine lettuce*
- *2 Tbs. coconut oil, melted*
- *1 tsp. sea salt*
- *½ tsp. fresh ground black pepper*
- *2 tsp. fresh grated parmesan*

## DIRECTIONS:

1. Heat grill on high.
2. Melt coconut oil.
3. Rinse romaine. Remove and discard any undesirable outer leaves.
4. Slice each head of romaine in half lengthwise.
5. On cut side, sprinkle oil, salt and pepper.
6. Reduce heat on grill to medium. Lay cut side of lettuce on grill for 2-3 minutes unti outside leaves are just wilted.
7. Remove to plate and top with parmesan.

**Serves 4**

# Spinach Salad

## INGREDIENTS:

- *8 cups organic baby spinach*

## OPTIONAL INGREDIENTS:

- *½ cup crumbled feta cheese or ¼ cup fresh grated parmesan*
- *6 kalamata olives, halved*
- *1 cup chopped cherry tomatoes*
- *Red bell pepper, sliced*
- *Green onions, sliced*
- *Mushrooms, sliced*
- *Avocado, cubed*
- *Carrots, diced*
- *Celery, diced*
- *Organic hard boiled egg, sliced*

## DRESSING INGREDIENTS:

- *3 Tbs. extra virgin olive oil*
- *1 Tbs. lemon juice*
- *½ Tbs. coconut aminos*
- *Sea salt*
- *Fresh ground pepper*

## DIRECTIONS:

1. Whisk together dressing ingredients.
2. Place spinach on plate. Add additional topping choices.
3. Drizzle dressing on top.

**Serves 4**

# Mexican Quinoa with Spinach

## INGREDIENTS:

- *1 ½ Tbsp. coconut oil*
- *1 medium onion*
- *2 cloves of garlic, minced*
- *1 jalapeno pepper, minced without seeds*
- *1 tsp. ground cumin*
- *1 tsp. ground coriander*
- *1 cup quinoa*
- *1 bell pepper, seeded and diced*
- *2 cups of vegetable stock or water*
- *Sea salt to taste*
- *2 cups fresh organic spinach, chopped*
- *2 tsp minced fresh parsley*

## DIRECTIONS:

1. Slice onion and mince garlic. Let sit for 5-10 minutes.
2. In a large saucepan, heat the oil and sauté the onion and jalapeno pepper with the cumin and coriander, until onion is almost translucent Add the garlic and sauté for another minute.
3. Add quinoa, bell pepper, stock and salt; cover and simmer for 10 minutes.
4. Add spinach, cover and simmer 5-10 minutes, or until liquid is absorbed.
5. Adjust seasoning as desired, stir in parsley and serve.

**Serves 4-6**

# Roasted Asparagus

## INGREDIENTS:

- *2 bunches asparagus*
- *1 Tbs. coconut oil*
- *Sea salt*
- *Fresh black pepper*

## DIRECTIONS:

1. Preheat oven to 450 degrees.
2. Wash asparagus and remove bottom woody part. Discard bottom part.
3. Melt coconut oil.
4. Place asparagus spears on cookie sheet. Brush coconut oil on asparagus. Sprinkle with salt and pepper.
5. Roast in oven for approximately 5 minutes or until tender. Watch carefully as they can quickly overcook and become brown.

Helpful Hint: To easily find the woody bottom part of the asparagus, bend about 2/3 of the way toward the lower end of the stalk. It will naturally snap at the tougher section. In a rush, snap one and then cut the rest to the same size; it will be close enough.

**Serves 4**

# Kale and Fruit Salad

## INGREDIENTS:

- *Yellow beet*
- *1 Tbs. of coconut oil*
- *Head of kale (any variety is fine, but I like Italian best)*
- *Juice of one lemon*
- *Extra virgin olive oil*
- *Kosher sea salt*
- *Raw, local honey*
- *Fresh ground black pepper*
- *Fruit of choice*
- *Additional vegetables of choice (optional)*
- *2 Tbs. - ¼ cup chopped almonds*

## DIRECTIONS:

1. Preheat oven to 450 degrees.
2. Using gloves, wash, peel and chop yellow beet into ½ inch cubes.
3. Place beet cubes in a small dish, add tablespoon of coconut oil and cook for 5 minutes. Stir beets to ensure coated in coconut oil. Continue cooking until just soft when speared with a fork, about another 10-15 minutes. Allow to cool.
4. De-stem kale, chop, rinse, and dry well.
5. Place kale in a bowl and toss with about 1/3 of the lemon juice, a drizzling of olive oil (about a half tablespoon) and sea salt. Massage kale for a few minutes until it starts to wilt. Set aside.
6. Wash, dry and slice fruit.
7. Thinly slice or grate any additional vegetables. Add vegetables to kale.
8. Make a dressing of remaining lemon juice, olive oil, honey, sea salt and pepper to taste.. Whisk well to emulsify.
9. Toss kale/vegetables with dressing and top with fruit, beets, and chopped almonds.

**HELPFUL HINT:** Although this recipe works well with any fruit, I think strawberries are the best combination. Purchase only organic strawberries though as non-organic strawberries have a high pesticide residue. Frozen and then thawed organic strawberries work well too.

**Serves 4**

# Sautéed Onions and Mushrooms

## INGREDIENTS:

- *1 medium onion*
- *2 ½ cups mushrooms*
- *1 Tbs. of ghee*
- *3 Tbs. vegetable broth*
- *Sea salt*
- *Fresh ground black pepper*

## DIRECTIONS:

1. Slice onion and allow to sit for 5-10 minutes.
2. Slice mushrooms
3. Heat ghee in skillet. Add onions and mushrooms. Sauté until tender.
4. If they begin to burn add vegetable broth and continue sautéing.
5. Season with salt and pepper to taste.

**Serves 4**

# Roasted Beets

## INGREDIENTS:

- One bunch beets (3 large or 6-8 small)
- 2 Tbs. of coconut oil
- Sea salt
- Fresh ground black pepper

## DIRECTIONS:

1. Preheat oven to 450 degrees.
2. Using gloves, wash, peel and chop large beets into ½ inch cubes. If using small beets there is no need to peel them.
3. Place beet cubes in a small dish, add oil and cook for 5 minutes. Stir beets to ensure coated in coconut oil. Continue cooking until just soft when speared with a fork, about another 10-15 minutes.
4. Season with salt and pepper to taste.

**Serves 4**

# Cabbage Salad

## INGREDIENTS:

- *4 cups Napa Cabbage, thinly sliced*
- *3 Tbs. extra virgin olive oil*
- *2 Tbs. rice vinegar*
- *1 tsp. coconut aminos*
- *1 Tbs. minced ginger*
- *1 medium clove garlic, pressed*
- *2 Tbs. chopped cilantro*

## DIRECTIONS:

1. Press garlic and allow to sit for 5-10 minutes.
2. Place cabbage on plate.
3. Whisk remaining ingredients together until well blended.
4. Drizzle dressing over cabbage.

**Serves 4**

# Roasted Vegetables

## INGREDIENTS:

- *1 zucchini*
- *1 cup squash*
- *1 red pepper*
- *1 yellow pepper*
- *1 lb fresh asparagus*
- *1 red onion*
- *2 Tbs. coconut oil*
- *1 tsp. sea salt*
- *½ tsp. fresh ground black pepper*

## DIRECTIONS:

1. Preheat oven to 450 degrees.
2. Cut all vegetables into bite sized pieces. Discard woody bottom pieces of asparagus.
3. Place in baking dish. Add coconut oil.
4. Cook for 5 minutes. Stir to ensure even coating of oil on all vegetables.
5. Roast for another 10-15 minutes, stirring occasionally, until vegetables are tender when speared with a fork.

**Serves 4**

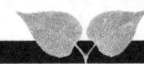

# desserts

# Almond Bars

## INGREDIENTS:

- *1 cup raw almonds*
- *1 Tbs. ginger root*
- *2 Tbs. sesame seeds*
- *1 cup raisins*
- *2 Tbs. raw honey*
- *½ scoop brown rice protein powder, approx. 3 Tbs.*

## DIRECTIONS:

1. Place all ingredients, except for honey, in a food processor and pulse until fairly fine but still having some texture (you don't want it to have the consistency of peanut butter).
2. Add honey and pulse just long enough for it to blend.
3. Press into a square about ¾ inch thick on a plate or square pan and refrigerate for about an hour or more.
4. Cut into 2 inch squares

**Serves 12**

# Chocolate Meringue Cookies

## INGREDIENTS:

- 3 egg whites, at room temperature
- ¼ cup raw honey or coconut sugar
- 6 squares of unsweetened chocolate, melted and cooled
- ½ tsp. of real vanilla extract

## DIRECTIONS:

1. Preheat oven to 350 degrees.
2. Line cookie sheets with parchment paper.
3. In a small mixer bowl, beat egg whites until very stiff.
4. Add honey or coconut sugar 1 tablespoon at a time, and continue beating until mixture is smooth and glossy and honey is completely incorporated.
5. Fold in chocolate and vanilla.
6. Drop by teaspoonfuls onto the cookie sheet.
7. Bake 15-18 minutes.

**HELPFUL HINT:** Choosing honey or coconut sugar is a matter of preference with this recipe. Honey will create a cookie that has a doughy texture in the middle. Coconut sugar will create a cookie that has crunchy pieces.

**Makes: about 48 cookies**

# Blueberry Ice

## INGREDIENTS:

- ½ cup frozen blueberries
- ½ cup coconut milk
- 2 Tbs. chopped almonds (optional)

## DIRECTIONS:

1. Place frozen blueberries in a bowl.
2. Top with coconut milk and allow to sit for 30 seconds.
3. Top with almonds if desired.

**Serves 1**

# Apple Treat

## INGREDIENTS:

- ½ apple
- 1 Tbs. almond butter
- ½ Tbs. raw honey
- ½ Tbs. hot water
- ½ Tbs. almonds, chopped
- ½ Tbs. unsweetened coconut

## DIRECTIONS:

1. In a small mixing bowl, blend the almond butter, honey, and water until smooth. It should be the consistency of caramel sauce.
2. Chop apple and place in bowl.
3. Drizzle sauce over the apple. Top with almonds and coconut.

**Serves 1**

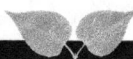

# RECIPE INDEX

## A
Aioli (Mayonnaise)................................. 43
Almond Bars ........................................ 117
Apple Treat ......................................... 120

## B
Baked Chicken  ..................................... 82
Baked Chicken Breast with Herbs ......... 78
Baked Cod............................................ 86
Balsamic Vinaigrette ........................... 40
Black Bean Hummus............................. 60
Blueberry Ice ...................................... 119
Boiled Spinach ..................................... 99
Breakfast Scramble.............................. 47

## C
Cabbage Salad ..................................... 112
Cabbage Spring Rolls ........................... 89
Caesar Salad ....................................... 100
Chef's Salad  ....................................... 73
Chicken Piquant  ................................. 88
Chicken Salad....................................... 67
Chocolate Meringue Cookies............... 118
Chopped Salad...................................... 69
Creamy Ginger Dressing ...................... 42
Curried Chicken Salad.......................... 71

## F
Fish in Parchment ................................ 84
Florida Rolls ........................................ 61

## G
Grilled Romaine................................... 105

## H
Huevos Rancheros ............................... 53

## K
Kale and Fruit Salad............................. 109
Kale Chips ............................................ 62

## L
Lemon Fish .......................................... 83
Lentils .................................................. 102
London Broil ......................................... 87

## M
Mashed Butternut Squash.................... 98
Mashed Cauliflower ............................ 104
Mexican Quinoa with Spinach ............ 107
Mexican Stuffed Chicken ..................... 85
Mini Quiche ......................................... 48
Morning Scramble ............................... 49
Mustard Chicken.................................. 80

## O
Orange Broccoli Chicken...................... 72

## P
Pickled Kale Salad ............................... 103
Puréed Beans........................................ 96

## Q
Quick Scallops...................................... 81

## R
Red Cabbage and Snow Pea Salad ..... 101
Red Pepper Hummus............................ 58
Red Pepper Vinaigrette........................ 41
Roasted Asparagus .............................. 108
Roasted Beets....................................... 111
Roasted Brussels Sprouts .................... 97
Roasted Vegetables ............................. 113

## S
Salmon in Orange Sauce...................... 77
Sautéed Onions and Mushrooms ....... 110
Shrimp Salad........................................ 70
Sirloin Steak......................................... 79
Spicy Breakfast Burrito ........................ 51
Spinach Frittata ................................... 50
Spinach Salad ...................................... 106
Steamed Vegetables............................ 95
Stuffed Tomato .................................... 68
Swiss Chard.......................................... 94

## T
Tangy Halibut....................................... 90
Trail Mix ............................................... 59
Turkey Wrap ........................................ 57

## V
Vegetable Omelet................................. 52

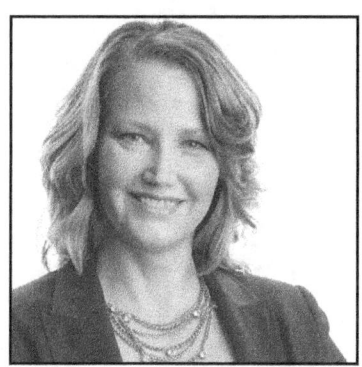

# About the Author

Kellie started her career in the world of non-profit and quickly found she could put the same number of hours in, working for herself, and make money. So she left to become an entrepreneur. With the purchase of her first location, she became the youngest female franchisee of 7-Eleven and soon afterward, she bought a second store. After five years, and meeting her husband-to-be, she sold her businesses and started in the McDonald's world. She worked her way up through the system, including Hamburger University, and ultimately became an approved franchisee. After ten years in the fast food industry she realized her continuous passion for healthy food was too incongruent with her career choice.

Kellie went back to school receiving a BS in Nutrition, Health and Wellness to add to her BA in Speech Communication. Wanting to find even healthier alternatives for teaching she received her Nutritional Therapy Practitioner degree the following year.

Kellie is the author of multiple books instructing how to use nutrient-dense whole foods to lose weight, improve health, and detoxify the body. She is the international radio show host of Eat Well to Live Well with Kellie Hill on Voice America every Monday at 2:00 p.m. Pacific. Find previous episodes at www.therightnutritionplan.com. Connect with Kellie on Facebook, Twitter, or Pinterest @The Right Plan, or via email at kellie@therightnutritionplan.com.

Years of working with private clients and instructing cooking classes lead Kellie to want to produce programs for individuals that didn't have the time, desire, or resources to be a private client. The 2 Week Weight Loss Program is one of the results.

www.ingramcontent.com/pod-product-compliance
Lightning Source LLC
Chambersburg PA
CBHW070151290526
45789CB00002B/720